WE'RE
PARENTS!

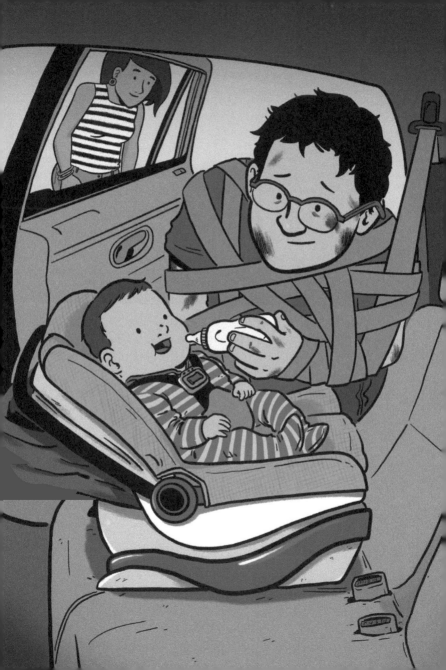

WE'RE PARENTS!

The New Dad's Guide to Baby's First Year

Everything You Need to Know to Survive and Thrive Together

ADRIAN KULP

Foreword by Jill Krause,
creator of *Baby Rabies*

Illustrations by Jeremy Nguyen

ROCKRIDGE
PRESS

For general information on our other products and services or to obtain technical support, please contact our Customer Care Department within the United States at (866) 744-2665, or outside the United States at (510) 253-0500.

Rockridge Press publishes its books in a variety of electronic and print formats. Some content that appears in print may not be available in electronic books, and vice versa.

Interior and Cover Designer: Antonio Valverde
Art Producer: Sue Bischofberger
Editor: Kim Suarez and Jesse Aylen
Production Editor: Andrew Yackira
Cover and interior illustration: © 2019 Jeremy Nguyen, except pp. 10-13.
Interior illustration: © 2019 Christian Dellavedova, pp. 10-13.

ISBN: Print 978-1-64152-415-5 | eBook 978-1-64152-416-2

For Ava, Charlie, Mason, Evelyn,
and my wife, Jen.

The road of parenting is certainly filled
with easy miles and beautiful moments,
but it's hitting those potholes together
that makes us family.

Contents

Foreword

What if I told you the biggest test of your life was something you could never ace, no matter how hard you studied? That you'll fail many times, even if you read every possible book and take thousands of pages of notes? But that you absolutely should still try anyway? Welcome to parenthood! It's the single most important thing you'll do, and one that you will never, *ever*, be perfect at.

I don't say that to scare you, but to encourage you to set your bar at ground level, and to commend you for picking up this book anyway. I think it's pretty common for parents to invest time learning all about pregnancy but, once the baby's here, some parents think the rest will work itself out. In reality, babies are much more mystical and confusing when they're finally outside the womb.

For my husband and I, our first parenthood year was an exhausted haze of wide-eyed stares, slow blinks, and sideways glances as we wondered *what was happening*? All of the anecdotal advice from well-meaning friends and family doesn't do enough to *actually* prepare you to be a parent of a baby in those first frazzled 12 months. But that's why Adrian wrote this invaluable guide.

We're Parents! is full of practical advice (high fives for our mutual dislike of baby shoes, Adrian), actionable steps for being an incredible, supportive partner, and a detailed path to guiding your baby through their healthy, happy first year. Along the way, you'll find checklists, check-ins, and the world's most epic collection of dad-worthy T-shirts.

Even if you still end up in public with explosive newborn poop running down the back of your backup shirt, you won't regret reading and preparing yourself for parenting during your baby's first year. There's no way to ace this, but showing up and trying counts a whole lot.

—Jill Krause, creator of *Baby Rabies*

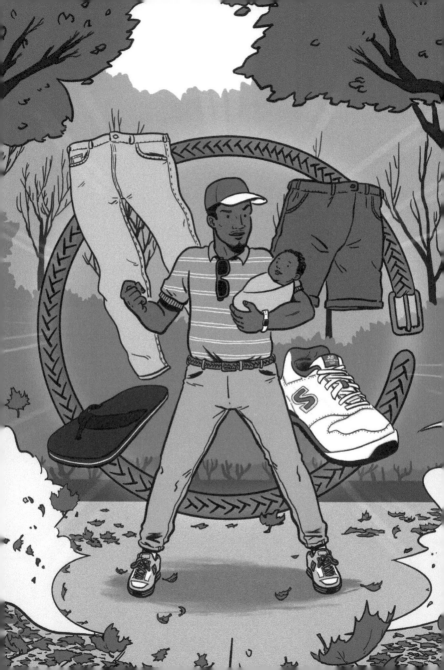

So You're a New Dad

It was a little over nine years ago, but I remember the moment with such clarity. Hearing my firstborn Ava's first breath and cry—this wasn't anything like the other "firsts" in my life. This didn't fall into the same category of hitting your first home run in youth baseball or nailing the elusive three-point turn on your driver's exam. This was a moment like no other.

I was experiencing a miracle, and it left me floating a hundred miles above the Earth. And at that moment it all began.

Those few hours after the birth, my wife and I felt like the center of the universe. It was like all of the Christmas mornings we've ever had, all rolled into one. We bonded together over the excitement and sheer joy that surrounded creating a life together. We were thrilled to introduce her to her grandparents and the family and friends who began trickling through the hospital door.

The morning after delivery? The novelty of living in the hospital had worn off completely. Sleeping on a cot with a paper pillow from the 1970s that held the scent of generations of fathers before me had become cringeworthy. Most hospitals don't really think about the partner's accommodations, and I soon found that when you're running on a severe lack of sleep, everything can start crashing around you.

This smack in the face was crisp and cold, but necessary. At the same time, I needed to find the levity in the situation or I was never going to survive.

Three days later we were released, and in the 24 hours after we left the hospital, I began to get the sense that *shit was getting real.*

In the hospital, everything is within arm's reach and you're confined to one room. They make those rooms so small on purpose, so you don't get too comfortable and want to stay with these on-call babysitters. Then you get home and all of a sudden it's "Where are the damn diapers?" or "Did I leave the wipes upstairs?" or even worse, "Did sleep deprivation just cause me to brush my teeth with Desitin?!"

That first night back in our apartment, without the hospital staff, I realized that we were it from here on out—just me, my wife, and this precious jewel. I had a decision to make. Sure, I could be a great assistant to my wife; I could play backup and do what was asked of me, like many other amazing fathers. But I wanted to be all in, and to completely rock at this.

As great as my intentions were, I was still wondering, "Where is the manual on what to do?" Yes, that stack of books that my wife had purchased was still sitting behind the toilet. But the idea of picking up those phone-book-thick texts felt more like studying for finals. I needed something easier—a kinder, gentler way to *quickly* learn what I should be doing and how I could step up and become the dad I knew I could be.

It was time to bring on the dad jeans, woven belts, and shorts that reveal too much upper-thigh hair. It was time to get equipped with the standard-issue white New Balance running shoes and prepare myself for the majestic "dad bod."

I was determined, for sure, but in those first few days after arriving home, I found myself questioning my every move. I was like a bomb tech assigned to disarm an explosive device, second-guessing which color wire I should cut. If I made the wrong move, was this device going to explode, covering me in baby vomit or sending fecal shrapnel onto my favorite T-shirt?

And these feelings of uncertainty didn't necessarily disappear right away. In fact, for weeks after the birth, as I walked around in broad daylight in public settings, I thought to myself, "Who in the hell gave me a kid? How am I responsible for something this fragile? This is the same guy that got his tongue pierced by a street vendor in Mexico on spring break—my judgment is questionable at best."

Having a baby was an event that took shots at me emotionally and physically, while challenging my confidence and self-esteem. But, within a few months, I had found a new comfort zone.

And in it all, my wife and I found our groove. We worked in tandem, and while it wasn't always pretty, easy, or neat, I can say that we did it together, and still do to this day. There are certainly times in which we operate as a physical team, but there are just as many times when one of us has to take the wheel while the other rests. There was never a shortage of desperate baby handoffs: "Tag! You're it."

I began to embrace the dad life. We decided that "one and done" wasn't for us. After Ava, we were blessed with two boys, Charlie and Mason. And not long after, during the course of writing the first book of the series, *We're Pregnant! The*

First-Time Dad's Pregnancy Handbook, we had Evelyn, the final joyful piece to our family puzzle.

As I write this, I'm actually living it for what (I think) will be the last time. With all those new dad experiences, I should be an ace, right? We'll see. The story is still being written, but I try to do my best every day.

First-Year Expectations

Now that your child is here, it's time to put in the hard work. And don't let anyone tell you that it's not hard. In fact, I'll tell you that every beautiful image that I posted on social media immediately following the birth of each of our four children captured a moment that never lasted more than 10 seconds.

When speaking to family, friends, or colleagues, I wanted all of them to feel like I was living in a heaven on earth. But while I was very happy, my cup simultaneously ran over with discontent, sleep deprivation, and anxiety over what the next day would bring. And in the world of picture-perfect parenting—or, as my wife calls it, the "Instagram side of life"—it can feel very lonely to see other people's perfectly filtered photos and imagine that everyone else has their shit under control. But dollars to donuts, I'm willing to bet that for every photo you see where things look easy, seamless, and calm, there are hundreds of moments full of thoughts like "What have we done?" Image crafting is great for artful food platters and home decor, but when it comes to parenting, everyone who's been there can see straight through the bullshit.

Of course, you're going to experience all of the great moments: the joy, the peace, the harmony. Those moments exist—but so do the chaos, the anxiety, and the sheer realness. And that's why I wrote this book.

At every pediatric appointment, the practitioner would turn to my wife and say "And how are *you* doing, Mom?" This is completely understandable. She'd been through a major surgery, her body and brain had been put through the wringer, and as every new parent knows, moms are all at risk for postpartum depression. As serious as my wife's recovery was, I have to admit: I felt alone, folks. My friends who had done this dad thing were busy with their own kids. I was worried that if I put a face to my emotions, people would call me immature or selfish, and so I kept my insecurities bottled up. But that wasn't a great plan, either.

I can now look back and say that becoming a dad comes with some hard truths that, once accepted, become easier to manage. Here are some tips for dealing with the learning curve:

TRY KEEPING UP. You'll have moments where a lightbulb flashes, and you think "I got this!" The reality is that just when you think you've got them figured out and mastered their current developmental state, babies hit you with a gut punch. They're crawling, they're cruising, they're chewing on a used Q-tip from the bathroom floor. And so you're off again, scrambling to keep up!

HONOR YOUR NEEDS. No one can bank sleep, but new parents often wish they'd taken the time to sleep in during the weeks leading up to delivery. Your body can survive with less than what you're giving it, but you also need to know when to take care of yourself. Sleep is important to being present as a father and a partner, so establish a plan before baby arrives so you can ensure that both of you get continuous sleep. And for the love of God, *sleep when your baby sleeps.*

SLOW DOWN YOUR JAM. Many men are patience deficient, including me. But pigs will fly sooner than you'll find a day when everything goes as planned. For your own sanity, lower your expectations—the world won't end because of a rogue bout of diarrhea. My wife and I have realized that when you plan for something to take longer, you're always on time, and with a newborn, that alone feels like a big win.

EVERY LITTLE THING COUNTS. Every little bit that you do for Team Family is worth it. Changing diapers, bouncing the baby or rocking her to sleep, taking on nighttime feedings, or even proactively packing the diaper bag can mean the world to your other half.

SHIT HAPPENS. And speaking of diaper bags, get ready for the onslaught. Be prepared to change a poop blowout (a veritable explosion that's come out the back, sides, or front of a diaper) at a moment's notice. Carry an extra outfit not only for your child, but also for yourself (I know, but trust me!). You'll get sick of turning your shirt inside out—most babies' bowel movements and urination are renowned for Olympian-level distance and speed.

CELEBRATE SMALL VICTORIES. Look for them everywhere—in a good nap, an uninterrupted dinner, even in a bath that doesn't include a baby peeing in your face.

FIND YOUR NEW NORMAL. Being home with a new baby is one of the most emotionally and physically taxing periods of your life. My wife and I had this idea that our babies would just naturally fit into our lives, and while that was solid mental preparation, we were wholly unprepared for how *messy* everything was those first weeks. But newborns will forgive a cluttered living room and dirty dishes in the sink, so you need to forgive yourself, too. You and your partner are going to have to figure out a new normal. Maybe it includes a lot of takeout and paper plates—and that's okay. Maybe laundry piles up and you pay the teenager down the street to fold it and find those orphaned socks. Work together, find your groove, and be a committed teammate. But above all else, remember that there's a difference between having a tough time and experiencing conditions like postpartum depression (page 7); this is a serious issue, and we'll talk about it more in chapter 1.

INVEST IN YOUR MARRIAGE (IT'S NEVER MATTERED MORE). It doesn't matter how strong of a bond you and your partner have, every relationship has a breaking point. Leave it to a newborn to find it and poke it. Someone once told us that couples therapy isn't for when you have a problem; it's to give you the tools to combat issues before they become problems. Issues that were present in your relationship are only going to be amplified tenfold after baby arrives. Conversely, if there are concerns lurking under the surface that you or your partner didn't want to deal with, baby's arrival will only bring them bubbling up. Some advice:

▸ Consider seeking couples therapy now in preparation for when things get difficult. This can be one of the best investments you make for your child—giving him a strong relationship to look up to and model his own after.

▸ Continue to "date" whenever you can, even if it's a picnic on the living room floor (my wife is a fan of Chinese food out of the containers and Netflix binges in bed).

▸ Try to find the humor in frustrating situations.

▸ Keep looking out for each other.

OWN YOUR MISTAKES. You're going to do things wrong or backward, or just plain make a bad decision, and it's going to be fine. Babies are pretty resilient. Just learn from your mistakes and move on.

Tag Team Partners

In the longer term, your team effort will hopefully mean nobody ever feels like they're going it alone. To that end, frequently assess to make sure that chores and childcare are shared—and yes, for us dads who work full-time, this also means *you*.

Think about this: Very shortly, life will return to *your* new normal, and you'll likely head back to work while Mom continues to heal and bond with baby. When you get home from a 10-hour workday, your partner has also been home working for 10 hours—and she didn't have her lunch break all to herself. Mom will not be able to function if she has the baby all day and all evening, and then is up with him all night, too. My wife would sometimes say, "I'm touched out." Having four kids, plus me, meant she was just tired of being touched, and as much as she thrives on having our children nearby, she also recognized that she needed a few minutes on her own to be still, for her own mental health. When either of us gets this tired, we have a cue for each other—it's generally putting a baby on the other's lap, followed by saying "Tag. You're it."

It's important to remember that "tag team" doesn't mean Mom is mentally responsible for keeping track of everything, and there are *lots* of things that need attention that first month: when did the baby last nurse/feed, how long, how much (if you're bottle-feeding), from what side (if baby's nursing), when was the last poopy diaper, when was the last nap, and on and on. If by the end of the day, all you've done was ask Mom what you need to do or expect her to proactively tell you, you're not playing an equal part of the team.

There will come a time that Dad also needs a break, and a happy, rested Mom can provide relief and support as well. You two have to stick together and communicate so nobody winds up crashing and burning.

Support Team

Dad is part of the nucleus, not the support system. No one can replace you, but the reality is that you're likely headed back to work fairly quickly after baby's birth. In this instance, help your partner round out the support system around the two of you to create the perfect team of people in your absence—whether it's friends, family, doulas, lactation consultants, or whomever (just not the neighbors from *Rosemary's Baby*!). The adage that it takes a village is true, and you and your partner will benefit greatly from having people you can rely on.

The advent of parenthood can be a true test of your relationship. There's no doubt about it, being in the trenches together for the first time is an ungodly amount of stress. You will both be exhausted, and initially just making it through a single hour, then the hours will become entire days. Some moments are going to require everything from both of you simultaneously, while other times you're going to become absolute winners at the tag team approach to parenting. This first part of this year is a time to be hyper self-aware and to focus on how you're communicating with your partner, how you're complementing each other, and how you can be the strengths to one another's weaknesses. Taking care of a newborn is a full-time job.

How to Use This Book

The beginning of this book focuses on what's known as the "fourth trimester." This time finds Mom recovering from childbirth, so we'll focus on how she's doing. But, after the first few weeks, she'll more than likely be mostly recovered from delivery and will be dealing with other changes. At that point, it's all about the tag team effort you'll put forth with your partner, and the year full of baby development and "firsts" you will celebrate together. This book isn't necessarily meant to be read from front to back in one sitting, but rather as a reference guide to make sure that you're keeping pace with your little one, or to obtain a dose of dad advice.

That said, this isn't a Dr. Spock book—this is an Adrian Kulp book. What I mean is, I am not a doctor—I'm a dad. And while this book explains what you can expect in the first year, this is based on real life. While I've offered a foundation of current research, what I find more valuable are the moments in which I can share my perspective on the miracles and challenges of parenthood, and the strategies that worked for us through that difficult territory of the first 12 months.

Tool Kits

Each chapter covers three months of development and includes a tool kit. Consider these tool kits your quick reference guides. These will include checklists of helpful things to do and look for, and I'll also offer tutorials and tips on skills you'll want to know and advice that can help at different stages. It's the real nitty-gritty, so I'll even tell you which baby gear's worth having, and which you can pass up.

Checklists

These checklists will serve as cheat sheets for things Dad needs to know for each month of that first year. New dads can quickly refer back to these after they've read the book; heck, you could even photocopy them and keep them in your back pocket or above the visor in your truck.

Tutorials and Tips

These tutorials are a combination of how-to advice, demos, and instruction. You may have learned some of these things—like how to swaddle or burp baby—in a parenting class, in the hospital, or even on YouTube. Hopefully these will serve as quick refreshers when all the knowledge has worn off, and you're in the midst of dealing with a screaming child, frantically trying to figure out why it's happening.

Baby Gear

When Jen and I had our first child, we spent hours wandering aisles of retail stores handcrafting a baby registry. We crowd-sourced social media for tips, advice, and suggestions on what we might need, so when the baby came, our apartment looked like Target's baby section had vomited across every square foot. The reality? We only used about 10 percent of our gear haul. My goal is to give you those must-haves based on our personal experience with four kids.

Monthly Stats

There's nothing worse than feeling uninformed, and in these early months, it can be helpful to get clues that help you under-stand what your partner or baby might be going through both physically and emotionally. During our first year as parents, I constantly felt like I was playing a guessing game, and I want to help you avoid that haze. In the early part of the book, these milestones will include observations about Mommy's physi-cal and mental recovery, and after the early months, much of the focus will shift to baby's developmental milestones. But I promise to keep reminding you about what your partner may need, too.

Monthly Goals

Similar to my first book, *We're Pregnant!*, I provide ideas for month-specific goals to help support your growing family. They'll be things Dad can focus on, and things you can focus on as a family unit. Goals are designed to help your baby thrive, but also to help your mind, body, and relationship in this strange new normal, so be sure to read these over—they can kick-start you in the right direction.

 STAFF MEETING Communication is key. These goals help you and your partner stay on the same page and communicate your needs to one another.

 HEALTH & WELLNESS These goals help you keep track of family needs when it comes to health care, nutrition, and overall wellness.

 PLAN AHEAD To ensure the best results or to prepare for the unexpected, planning ahead is vital. These goals ensure you're one step ahead.

 CRUISE DIRECTOR Dads can be fun and organized! These goals will suggest activities to do together as a family, or in playgroups with fellow new parents and their babies.

 SELF-CARE Just like Mom, Dad needs to recharge so he can be the best version of himself for his family. These goals offer a chance for Dad to take much-needed breaks.

DADDY DOULA Being in touch with Mom's postpartum needs is an essential gift to your family. These goals will offer ways Dad can support Mom's health and happiness during the postpartum period.

 BONDING TIME These suggestions include some of my favorite things to do to solidify the bond with both baby and Mom.

 MR. FIX-IT These goals involve things Dad can do to help with maintenance and cleaning.

BROWNIE POINTS These goals are thoughtful everyday touchstones to show your partner how highly you value her well-being and your relationship.

Securing the Foundation

As you start this new adventure, it may feel like there's so much to learn—and there is! But you'll do it all together—the diapers, the bottles, the baths. Parenthood can be an isolating experience; your entire life has shifted gears in order to meet the 24/7 needs of your new baby. "Nightlife" takes on a whole new meaning. But this is where you and your partner can find comfort: in each other.

All bets are off the first few weeks—you may find yourself eating cold pizza over the sink for breakfast. You are, at this point, surviving. But after a few hundred rounds of diapers, bottles, and baths, you're going to realize you're getting the hang of this and might actually be getting good at it. By keeping at it, you and your partner will develop a groove, and one day you'll realize you're having fun with all this, and that's one of those lightning-strike moments. Congratulations, new dad—you're no longer just surviving; you're actually thriving. Now, let's get you there.

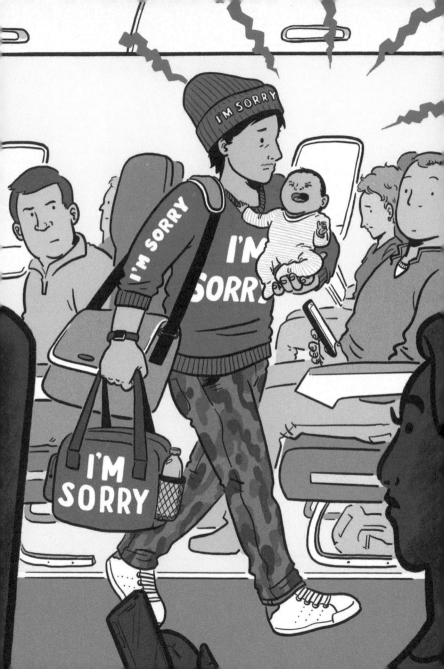

CHAPTER ONE

0 TO 3 MONTHS

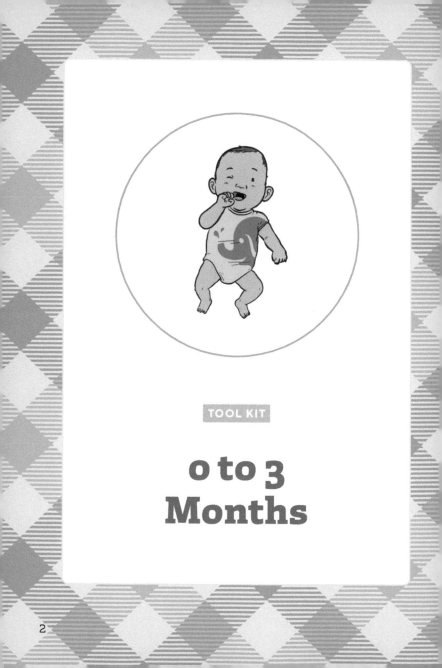

0 TO 3 MONTH CHECKLIST

HOME

☐ Make sure your home is free of lead-based paints, asbestos, and any type of insect infestation.

☐ Begin to introduce pets to the new baby (see page 20).

☐ Begin building a babysitter/support system schedule. Consider those who can help during the week, in the evenings, and on weekends.

☐ Set up the nursery: assemble furniture and baby gear, and install curtains or blinds that block sunlight.

☐ Set up the baby monitor.

☐ Establish a strategy for visitors (see page 6).

☐ Make a meal plan and a household chore plan.

BABY

MONTH 1

☐ Watch for jaundice in the first few days. If baby appears yellowish, even in the whites of her eyes, let the doctor know. This common condition responds to sunlight exposure or light therapy treatment.

☐ Spend as much time as possible just enjoying these first moments together. Touch baby often: massage him, cuddle him, gently move his legs in a cycling motion.

☐ Support baby's neck whenever you hold her.

☐ At nighttime, keep lights low and activity to a minimum.

- ☐ Keep the umbilical site clean and dry and keep the circumcision site clean (if applicable).
- ☐ Be careful with the fontanel (soft spot) on baby's head.
- ☐ When changing diapers, wipe the baby from front to back.
- ☐ Try to keep breast milk as the baby's main food source for the first 6 months, and up to 12 if possible. If not, invest in a good organic formula—buying in bulk saves money!

MONTH 2

- ☐ Put baby into her crib when she's still drowsy, so she can learn to fall asleep by herself.
- ☐ Speak to your baby often. She loves the sound of your voice.
- ☐ Give baby plenty of opportunities to move and assume different positions.
- ☐ Continue learning what your baby likes and what soothes him.

MONTH 3

- ☐ Start tummy time. Some babies find this frustrating at first, but it's so good for them and helps them get stronger. Look up fun tummy-time activities to get ideas that work for your baby.
- ☐ When baby wakes up crying, resist the urge to run in. Give him a few minutes to try to soothe himself back to sleep.
- ☐ Provide lots of colorful visual stimuli for baby to enjoy.

☐ Continue chatting up your baby. This helps develop her own communication skills—she may even begin to respond in different ways.

MOM

☐ If breastfeeding is an issue, contact a lactation specialist.

☐ Mom should be eating well and drinking lots of water, especially (but not only) if she's nursing.

☐ Take stock of Mom's emotional well-being. Mood swings can be attributable to changing hormones, but you'll want to be watchful for signs of postpartum mood disorders like anxiety and depression (page 7).

MEDICAL APPOINTMENTS

☐ Schedule your first pediatrician appointments.

☐ Obtain and review baby's vaccination schedule.

☐ Begin a list of questions for the doctor (those that can wait until the appointment).

EVENTS

☐ Schedule a newborn photo shoot.

☐ Send out birth announcements.

☐ Begin investigating and planning any relevant ceremonies related to your baby's birth (bris, baptism, etc.).

Tips & Tutorials

Quality of Life / Survival

HOW TO BE AN EFFECTIVE GATEKEEPER

Whether it's your baby's loving Grandma or a neighbor visiting, you can be the hero of the moment by speaking up for your partner and her needs.

In the hospital, we welcomed everyone—but that's only because my wife and I discussed it in advance and it was what we wanted. Many hospitals have an open-door policy, which can be nice, but it leaves room for the overstayer who brings their restless 4-year-old (who wants to writhe around on the hospital bed). This can be your first "bad guy" role: "Mom's getting tired. It's probably best to let her get some rest now. Thank you so much for coming." If it becomes an issue, sneak out and enlist a hospital staff member to come and tell your guests that it's time for vitals.

Once you're back home, work together to decide when visits should be scheduled, and how long they will last. If someone shows up unannounced, it's okay to start putting a note on the door or say, "We've had a long night. Can we take a rain check?" Your family's wellness comes first.

The next gate you're protecting is baby's. Only the closest family and friends really need to be holding the baby. My wife and I always felt like the more people to love on our little ones, the better. But the reality is that with more people come more germs. Our pediatrician recommended that everyone wash and sanitize their hands beforehand and use a barrier between the baby and their clothing, like a blanket or burp pad. No one aside from the two of you ever needs to touch baby's face or hands. Just remember: if you're not comfortable, just kindly say you're waiting until the baby is a bit older.

The final gate is the back door. Have a code between you and your partner. If Mom winks at you, it's time to wrap up this visit. Announce that Mom's exhausted and offer to walk your visitor to their car for a nice send-off.

KNOWING THE SIGNS OF POSTPARTUM MOOD DISORDERS

"Postpartum depression" has become the umbrella term for mood disorders that new moms experience due to a combination of factors, such as fluctuating hormones, high stress levels, sleep deprivation, and exhaustion. Women may also experience the more common but lesser-known postpartum anxiety. Certainly, childbirth can set hormones and emotions loose all over the place, so a little crying and worrying is to be expected. But when is it just the "baby blues," and when has it crossed the threshold into something more serious? There's a litany of research on the subject, but here's the short version.

▸ "Baby blues" are characterized by temporary symptoms such as mood swings, crying, anxiety, feeling overwhelmed, irritability, difficulty concentrating, and difficulty sleeping that all usually subside within about 2 weeks.

- Postpartum depression or anxiety can last for months, or longer if not treated.

- Dads experience postpartum depression, too.

- Postpartum depression is temporary and very treatable.

Signs and symptoms vary but can include the following:

- Excessive crying

- Rage or anger

- Severe mood swings

- Difficulty bonding with baby

- Severe fatigue or restlessness

- Withdrawal from others

- Feelings of despair, hopelessness, guilt, or unworthiness

- Feelings that you're not a good parent

- Difficulty concentrating or making decisions

- Diminished interest in activities

More severe symptoms such as hallucinations may be a sign of postpartum psychosis.

If you suspect that you or your partner may be experiencing any of these symptoms, talk to your health care provider and contact a support group such as Postpartum Support International at 1-800-944-4773. For emergencies, call 911 or a suicide hotline like the National Suicide Prevention Lifeline at 1-800-273-8255 (see Resources, page 184) right away. **The most important thing to remember is that these feelings are temporary and treatable.**

Eat

HOW TO BOTTLE-FEED

You and the little one are all alone and it's time to bottle-feed? You've got this.

1. **SET UP THE BOTTLE**. Grab a clean bottle, nipple, and seal. Pour in the formula or breast milk and seal it, tipping to make sure it's a tight seal.

2. **WARM THE BOTTLE.** Set the bottle in a bottle warmer or a pot of warm water for a few minutes. (Note that glass bottles can heat up quickly while the milk inside will still be cold. Plastic seemed to show a cooler exterior temperature and warmer fluid.)

3. **TEST THE TEMPERATURE**. Before you feed, *always* test the milk on your wrists before giving it to your baby. The perfect temperature is if you cannot feel it at all. If it seems too warm for you, it's definitely too warm for him.

4. **POSITION BABY.** Lay baby in a reclining position in your arms, hold the bottle in an upright position with the nipple touching his mouth. He will know what to do.

Insert the nipple to a point that baby is sucking comfortably, then cuddle in and enjoy the experience. Sometimes this will take a drop or two of breast milk or formula on the lips for the baby to gain interest.

5. BURP BABY. When he takes a break, burp him about halfway through the feeding.

HOW TO PROPERLY BURP BABY

1. Hold baby against your chest with his chin on your shoulder and gently pat his back using a cupped hand.

2. Seating your baby on your knee, supporting his neck and chest with your hand, gently pat his back with your other cupped hand. You may or may not get a burp (a satisfying achievement!).

3. Laying your baby across your knee, supporting his head, neck, and chest with your hand, gently pat his back using a cupped hand.

Soothe

HOW TO READ BABY'S CUES

There are a few key, seemingly subtle, cues that your baby
sends to let you know what she needs. Crying is usually the last
and final cue. Before baby starts to cry and gets to the point of
no return, know what to look for. It can mean the difference
between a peaceful transition or an all-out cry fest. Here are the
essential baby cues to know.

HUNGER

Early cues

Stirring   Mouth opening   Turning head
Seeking/rooting

Mid cues (a.k.a. Feed me, *now*!)

Stretching   Increased movement   Putting hand
to mouth

Late cues

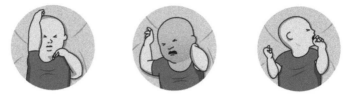

| Agitated | Turning red | Crying |

* If you miss the earlier cues, you might need to calm and soothe baby first before feeding. See below for more tips and details.

TIRED/SLEEPY

▶ Yawning

▶ Rubbing eyes

▶ Pulling ears

▶ Clenched fists

▶ Losing interest in
  things and people

NEEDS A CHANGE OF SCENERY

▶ Losing eye contact

▶ Squirming or kicking

PARENTING HACK TIP

If you missed the earlier cues and need to soothe baby first, here are some tips and suggestions.

▶ Swaddling baby

▶ Rocking him

▶ Offering skin-to-skin contact

▶ Stroking baby's skin lightly

▶ Talking to baby

HOW TO SWADDLE BABY

Want to find baby's cozy place? Swaddle her. It's like folding a burrito:

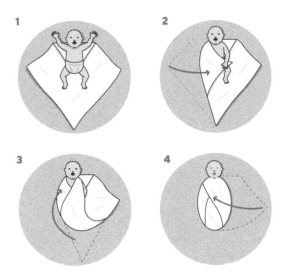

1. Fold the top edge of the swaddle blanket in. Lay the baby with her head at the fold.

2. Bring the right corner to the left and tuck it under the baby.

3. Then bring the bottom up and tuck it into the first fold.

4. Finally, bring the left corner to the right and wrap around. Only the baby's head and neck should be exposed. The swaddle should be snug but not too tight—she should be able to move her hips and knees.

Sleep

SUDDEN INFANT DEATH SYNDROME (SIDS) AWARENESS

Every parent thinks about it, and as a fellow parent, I want you to know this worry is natural—dare I say, it's the first of many issues you will worry about. There are a few preexisting conditions that can increase the risk, but here's what you should know that can help.

BABY SHOULD SLEEP BY HIS PARENTS. According to the American Academy of Pediatrics, babies should sleep in the same room as their parents for at least 6 months in their own crib, bassinet, or co-sleeper. There is significant research that says sharing a room with Mom and Dad can lower a baby's risk of SIDS by as much as 50 percent.

BABY SHOULD SLEEP ON HER BACK. SIDS is more common in babies who sleep on their belly or side. For the first year, encourage belly-up, back-down sleep.

FIRM SURFACES ARE BEST. Fluffy comforters, waterbeds, and pillows seem cozy, but they can block baby's airway.

CO-SLEEP WITH BABY IN A SAFE SPACE. While my wife and I have been big fans of co-sleeping, if you are going to co-sleep make sure you use a bed insert that allows baby to have his own safe space.

DON'T OVERHEAT BABY. While it's tempting to bump up the heat for the baby, being too warm can increase the risk of SIDS.

Other factors that increase the risk include exposure to secondhand smoke, low birth weight, brain defects, and respiratory issues.

HOW TO FIND A BEDTIME ROUTINE

Establishing a routine has many benefits: It helps baby know when naptime's coming and helps him fall asleep quicker, sets a family routine, and helps baby associate bedtime with the comfort of bonding. All of this makes for a happy, well-rested baby.

Here are some tips to set a routine into motion.

MAKE A PLAN. Giving a bath or massage, snuggling, reading a book together, singing gentle songs, and lowering the lights all set the stage for downtime. Find your groove and enjoy this unrushed time together.

READ THE SIGNS. When you catch on to your baby's sleepy cues, you'll be able to time naps for when they make the most sense. This timing can help you establish a routine.

FINISH IN THE CRIB. When baby is drowsy, move her to the crib so she can learn to fall asleep on her own. Keep trying, even if you don't succeed at first. This is a major win—it will set her up for good sleep habits going forward.

AIM FOR CONSISTENCY. Although life happens, try to keep the routine and timing regular to help baby know what to expect. Now the challenge is to work your family's life around your newest member's routine!

RESUME LIFE. Don't feel like you need to tiptoe around while baby naps. One of my greatest accomplishments is vacuuming during naptime—my kids can now sleep through anything.

Learn and Play

HOW TO PLAY WITH YOUR NEWBORN

It may be too early to register for T-ball, but you can still have fun with your new baby.

WORK THOSE LEGS. I used to lay my little ones on a blanket and work those arms and gams—up and down, or bicycle motion, gently.

ENGAGE THE SENSES.

- ▶ **Sound:** Your voice is the best entertainment baby can ask for. Sing to them. Confide in them. Let's be honest, it's cheaper than therapy. I always found myself talking to our babies like I would talk to my drunk college roommate as I maneuvered him back home: "You're a big walker and talker now, aren't you?" In addition to the unexpected entertainment value, your voice can help them pick up words and tone at an early age.

- ▶ **Sight:** By 1 month old, baby can make eye contact and focus on things about a foot away. Entertain baby—and yourself—by making faces. Shake a rattle and see if baby can find the source of that noise. Play Follow the Finger—as your baby's vision continues to sharpen, spending a few minutes playing "tracking" games will speed the process.

▶ **Touch:** Offer soft, gentle massage. Caress his cheek with a silk blanket or a stuffed animal. Touch his feet in rhythm with a song.

Clean

HOW TO GIVE BABY A BATH

Whether you use a fancy tub insert, a stand-alone infant bath, or the kitchen sink, you'll want to prepare your work space.

Gather the following:

▶ Gentle baby soap

▶ Two or three washcloths

▶ Plastic cup

▶ Soft baby towel and a thick plush towel

▶ Clean outfit (for baby, although you may need a clean shirt, too, when all is done)

It's now time for a bath!

1. **SET UP A LANDING AREA.** Clear an area and spread a towel over another thick plush towel.

2. **BEWARE OF THE BELLY BUTTON.** If baby has not yet lost his umbilical cord stump, give baby a head-to-toe sponge bath with a warm, damp washcloth with a little baby soap, avoiding the belly button. Wash baby's bottom last, then set that washcloth aside. Rinse off any soap with the second warm, wet washcloth. Wrap baby in the towel.

3. **FILL THE BATH.** If the umbilical cord stump is gone, you can fill the bath halfway, just enough for baby to sit in some warm water. Test the water before placing baby in the bath. Never take your hand off baby.

4. **WASH HEAD TO TOE.** Starting with baby's head, use a warm, damp washcloth to lather a small amount of soap onto his skin. Support baby's body and neck as you work your way down, and save baby's bottom for last. Set that washcloth aside—it's done.

5. **RINSE.** Fill the plastic cup with water from the bath and pour it over the baby's trunk and legs to keep him warm and rinse him. Wet the second washcloth and wash the soap out of his hair.

6. **WRAP UP.** Lay baby on the towel. Wrap your bundle in the clean towel, spot-drying his head and body. Hug baby until he's warm and dry, and then change him into his clean outfit.

I have to take this opportunity to share a few PSAs, even though many of these are common sense. Don't use a sink with a garbage disposal in it. Don't leave baby unattended for even a split second. Baby is slippery. And baby may pee. You can use a third washcloth to keep this area covered while you bathe him, so *you* do not get a bath. Additionally, my wife loves to bathe with our infants, and considers it some of the best bonding time.

HOW TO HANDLE CIRCUMCISION

If you've decided to circumcise your baby boy, you'll need to know your aftercare. A baby boy's circumcision normally heals within 7 to 10 days. During this time, when changing diapers, you'll want to delicately remove any poop or mess with a warm, damp cloth. Keep Vaseline or some type of barrier cream as recommended by your pediatrician on it at all times so that the wound doesn't get stuck to the diaper and to avoid penile adhesion (when the wound sticks to the penis itself). Your pediatrician may direct you to cover the cream with a piece of sterile gauze to protect the site.

PARENTING HACK TIP

Stock up on onesies with the envelope-looking top. It's actually a term for a functional onesie with a folded neckline that can be pulled down over the baby instead of up. In the event of a blowout, it saves you the agony of having to drag feces across your child's face. (And it should be noted that it took three kids for me to figure this one out.)

Babyproof

KEEPING AN IMMOBILE INFANT SAFE

At this stage, you're not really babyproofing, but you can ensure that baby's environment is safe. This may include:

- ▶ Ensuring that baby's sleeping arrangements meet with current safety standards (see page 14).

- ▶ Making sure that an adult is always present when your baby and pets are in the same room (see How to Introduce Pets below). The same logic applies to toddlers. Pets and toddlers can both behave in unpredictable ways.

- ▶ Being watchful that the room temperature is not overly warm or cold and that baby is dressed appropriately for the temperature.

HOW TO INTRODUCE PETS

Your pet was your original baby, and now there's a new star in town. What's poor Cooper the Boston terrier to think? To set yourself and your pet up for success, consider these tips.

START EARLY. If you're reading this in advance of baby's arrival, you can introduce gates to your pet now. Let them smell the baby creams and diapers so they become familiar with their scents. Buy them a new doggie or kitty bed to replace their former spot between you and your partner. If baby's already here, looks like it's time for introductions.

INTRODUCE SLOWLY. When Ava was born, I brought home a wet diaper from the hospital for the dog to sniff before we were discharged so that he was familiar with her scent. When baby comes home, take your time with introductions. Try not to scold your pet every time they go near the baby. Make efforts to resume normal life and allow your pet to do the things they've always done. If your pet gets overly rambunctious in baby's presence, rather than banishing the dog, try handing off baby to someone else and giving your pup a squeeze for a few minutes.

KEEP THE LOVE ALIVE. As time-challenged as you may be, try to carve out moments to love your pet and let them know they still matter. If you can, enlist friends, neighbors, or a dog walker to help fill in the gaps.

BE WATCHFUL. Don't leave pets and infants alone together. Sudden baby movements or noises can startle pets, and animals are animals—even the best of them can behave in unpredictable ways.

Pediatric

KNOW WHEN TO CALL THE DOC

Common baby ailments include colic, thrush, diaper rash, cradle cap, baby acne, clogged tear ducts, increased or decreased urination or bowel movements—the list goes on—and that's not even including illnesses such as fevers or colds. As a parent, you are now charged with the well-being of someone else. So when do you call the doctor? Here are some considerations:

DON'T WAIT. Fever, extended bouts of crying, vomiting—some signs clearly point to calling the doctor. Don't wait the weekend—get help, even if it means a trip to the ER.

TRUST YOUR GUT. What about that gray area? Maybe you're not sure. Trust your gut. When there's any doubt, call the doctor. You are the parents, and your instincts are reliable. You chose this professional to respond to your baby's needs, and as such, you have every right to seek their medical opinion.

FIND THE RIGHT FIT. If you find that the doctor is less than responsive, patient, and/or helpful, you might want to consider asking around about a more accessible pediatrician.

Baby Gear

Must-Have

▸ **Cloth and/or regular diapers:** This is a big decision. One is perhaps more environmentally conscious and the other not so much, but saves time. We tried using cloth diapers, but it just wasn't for us. My wife and I put disposables on our registry with our later kids. We stored cases in the laundry room, which served as an emergency stash.

▸ **Bottles:** Plastic bottles are generally cheaper than glass; however, they also can potentially leach chemicals into breast milk or formula during the warming process. If you want to go plastic, heat the liquid *before* putting it into the bottle. Glass bottles are heavier and, of course, be sure not to drop them.

▸ **Co-sleeper or side-sleeper bassinet:** Summer and SwaddleMe make great versions of the middle-of-the-bed option, and Arm's Reach makes a version of a co-sleeper that pulls up next to the bed, making late-night in-and-out easy. Remember that baby has been inside Mom's tummy for the better part of a year; expecting baby to dive headfirst into a crib with no one in the room is a difficult ask for a newborn. Plus, research supports the idea that babies who sleep near their parents are connected to their breathing rhythms. This can be very beneficial for baby, and something to keep in mind in regard to SIDS (see page 14).

▶ **Breast pump and accessories:** You can use the motorized pump version that comes in a nifty carrying case (we were always partial to the Medela brand). But Dr. Brown sent my wife a hand expresser that came in "handy" in times of engorgement when the baby wasn't willing or able to nurse. My wife swears that for minimal pumping, the manual pump has been far better for her than any electric one.

▶ **Diaper bag:** You can find a million of these online marketed specifically toward dads, which is awesome. I use a backpack with plenty of carabiner loops and side pouches for bottles or liquids.

▶ **Changing pad:** Something that resists stains and liquids and offers a bit of cushion will help on those days at the playground when you need to set up a diaper station triage on a hot park bench.

▶ **Plastic bags:** You never know when you're going to need to tie up a blowout or the clothes baby was wearing at the time.

▶ **Burp cloths:** These are good to keep handy if you don't want to burn through T-shirts at a daily rate. In fact, I've actually used those soiled T-shirts as future burping pads to save the next generation of Hanes V-necks.

- **Sun protection accessories:** Fresh air is wonderful, but do everything you can to keep baby out of direct sunlight. Their skin is very sensitive, and they can't use sunscreen for the first 3 months or so. You will want to have a shade on your stroller and a sun umbrella if you have to be out at the height of the day. Also consider a battery operated or rechargeable fan that clips on to the stroller.

- **Baby car seat:** For kids this age, choose a rear-facing car seat. Leave the convertible seats for when they are past age 2.

- **Stroller:** We use a quick Snap-N-Go style, which is a stroller frame you can snap the car seat right down into (this will come in handy because you won't want to wake baby up to get him in and out of the vehicle and into a stroller).

- **Baby carrier:** Years ago, I added the baby carrier to our registry, along with an exterior pack (worn on the back) for hikes, etc. Both came in extremely handy, and if I hadn't been able to wear my kid, I would've accomplished virtually *nothing* in those first few years.

- **Protective ointment:** Try A&D, Vaseline, Desitin, Balmex, Triple Paste, Boudreaux's Butt Paste, Aquaphor, or Calmoseptine—you'll find your favorite. Barrier creams for preventing rashes look clear, while thicker white pastes are generally for treating diaper rashes.

Nice to Have

▶ **Baby apps:** There are a lot of great baby apps out there. We used the Wonder Weeks app, which laid out developmental milestones based on due date rather than birth date. It will tell you what's ahead, what developmental milestones to look out for, and what fun and engaging elements to expect during the next couple of weeks.

▶ **Mirror:** Some sources argue that they're not safe because they encourage taking your eyes off the road, but I feel that a mirror for the opposite side of the car seat is crucial when you're driving by yourself, so you can see into your rearview mirror and quickly confirm that your baby isn't in distress. A mirror also comes in handy as an attachment within baby's crib—seeing themselves can occupy them long enough for you to get a few pieces of laundry folded.

▶ **Bottle warmer:** By the time I needed a warm bottle, I didn't have the luxury of firing up a device, adding water, and waiting until it reached the desired temperature. If you're using formula and have the option, buy one of those amazing Keurig-style machines that both heat and dispense formula.

▶ **Stationary swing:** It's nice to be able to put baby down where he'll be happy for a while. We have enjoyed two kinds of swings: a traditional baby swing and a bouncer-style swing.

- **Mobile:** You can find the most amazing handcrafted mobiles on Etsy, and there are retail outlets that offer a product that serves the same purpose. Anything that can hang from the ceiling with highly contrasting colors and patterns is great to keep their attention, even if it's a collection of your favorite beer cans (although I recommend empty cans).

- **Pacifier:** I could go either way on this one. Some of our kids loved their pacifiers because they provided an opportunity for them to self-soothe. The downside is that toddlers can become addicted to the "binky," and breaking the habit can be challenging. My advice? Do what works for now—don't stress over this one.

- **Rattles:** These encourage sensory development and can distract fussy babies.

- **Teething toys:** Babies love to chew. Be conscious about the kind you buy—BPA-free claims aren't always reliable. Choose those specifically designed for chewing enjoyment. Wooden ones are actually a smart choice, as are ones you can refrigerate.

- **Play mat:** We've had the same baby play mat for all our kids—a simple mat with two arches that rise over baby with hanging toys and mirrors.

- **Jogging stroller:** Getting outside is important—take it from someone who nearly became an agoraphobe after the birth of our first child.

Pass

▶ **Wipe warmer:** These were introduced to the market after we started having kids, and I felt like I could save myself some cash by simply crunching that wipe in my warm fist for 20 seconds. Confirmed. Plus, this gadget tends to dry out the wipes.

▶ **Changing table:** With full supervision, virtually anything can be a changing table if you lay a changing pad on it. And unless you are a real stickler, a dedicated changing table will quickly be covered with folded laundry, diapers, papers, and baby lotions, leaving no room to lay baby on it.

▶ **Crib bedding:** With current safety guidelines dictating nothing in the crib except the sheet and a bed skirt, the former bumpers, comforters, and wedges are more than just unnecessary—they can be dangerous.

▶ **Shoes:** I get it. Some people go wild over shoes, and I will never convince them not to buy shoes for their 2-week-old baby. But if you aren't that person, why not just let them enjoy life in socks for a while? I've found our kids start wearing soft shoes around 1 year old.

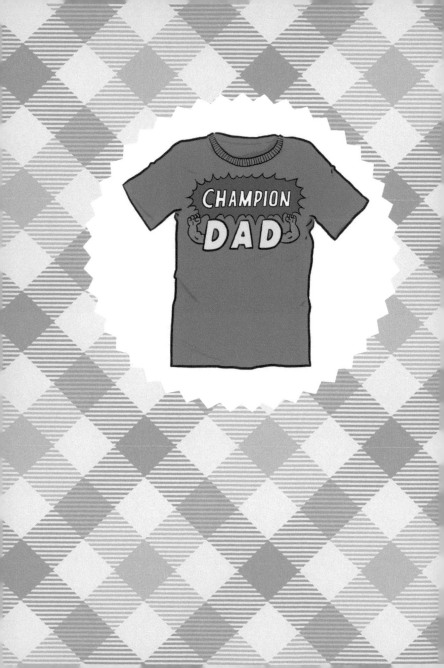

MONTH 1

AVERAGE SIZE	WEIGHT COMPARISON
7 pounds	6-foot aluminum stepladder, gallon of paint

How was that drive home from the hospital? Did you have your hands at 10 and 2 for the first time ever, white-knuckling the wheel? Not since my days in college, when I was assigned the job of keg deliveryman during a snowstorm, have I felt such overwhelming pressure to safely deliver a package.

So, you got home in one piece, and the comforts of your own surroundings are amazing: not having hospital staff (awesomely helpful as they may be) in and out of your room every five minutes, and not having to sleep on a reclining chair with more miles on it than a motel bed.

But along with all those nurse visits came a ton of help: a literal Bible of knowledge at your beck and call. I tried to follow their every move; they are essentially showing you the ropes in keeping your baby alive, skipping the midterms and sending you right to the final exam. And as soon as you step one foot outside that hospital, it's all on you and your partner.

Hopefully during this time you have a ton of support: the pediatrician, grandparents, a hospital lactation consultant, possibly your doula. Or maybe it's just you. Either way, the first few weeks are exciting but stressful. One thing the nurses told me really stuck: *If you can just begin by mimicking the hospital routine at home, you've already conquered the most important part of the transition.*

The nursing and feeding schedules will really stay the same, with minor adjustments from day to day. And babies will poop. And yes, nighttime is going to suck.

So prepare for the first week or so to be very draining physically, mentally, and emotionally. But at the end of every day, just remember that there most definitely is a light at the end of the tunnel.

Every man before you (okay fine, *most* men—we have lost a few soldiers along the way) got through this and many went on to have one, two, three, or, in the case of reality patriarch Jim Bob Duggar, 18 more children. It *will* get better. Life *will* become easier. You and your partner *will* find a way for this to work for both of you.

My most simplified advice during the first week is this: Don't count on getting the rest you need, nor the rest you're accustomed to. Counter that by lowering your expectations of yourself in these exhausted moments. Strong will. Strong coffee. Nap when baby naps.

MOM STATS

▶ Whether it was a natural birth or a C-section, Mom is in recovery mode and will be bleeding heavily for anywhere from 1 to 4 weeks postpartum.

▶ We know it goes without saying, but we're going to say it anyway: sex is off-limits this month.

▶ Hormones are adjusting and emotions are potentially running high—this can include crying, feelings of frustration, and anxiety.

▶ Breastfeeding may be taking its toll on Mom, as she's dealing with depleted nutrients and having baby attached to her 24/7.

▶ Nursing blisters may pop up (ouch!). Epsom salt baths can open up Mom's ducts and promote more free flow, and so can resting on all fours and dangling her breasts like in downward dog (no lie).

▶ Postpartum depression can occur in Mom and even Dad—this is different from baby blues (see page 7) and should be addressed immediately with your family doctor.

BABY STATS

▶ Most children will lose one-tenth of their birth weight in the first week, but will regain it in the 2 weeks that follow. If they don't, your pediatrician will talk you through some options for helping baby gain weight faster.

▶ Some babies might have a cone shape to their skull from birth. Don't worry, this flexible shape is perfectly normal and baby's head will begin to reshape on its own.

▶ Baby will tire easily—sucking while nursing while breathing is a complex maneuver for newborns.

▶ The fetal position becomes less and less pronounced; babies begin to stretch their arms and legs.

▶ Baby's excrement will transition from black tar (meconium) to liquid charcoal to various blends of mustard and eventually a solid Dijon, where it will happily stay until you start her on solid food.

▶ Be hyperaware of the soft spot on top of baby's head, also called the fontanel.

▶ Crying is going to happen—get comfortable letting baby go for 2 to 5 minutes.

▶ Colic is real, though it is somewhat of a mystery and has few to no symptoms. Look for the threes: any healthy baby that cries for more than 3 hours a day, 3 days a week for more than 3 months. Look into gripe water, probiotics, and herbs (no, not marijuana)—check with your pediatrician for some ideas to ease baby's (and your) pain.

▶ Cradle cap (white or yellow scales on baby's scalp) and baby acne are not dangerous and will go away after a few weeks with mild shampooing.

▶ Keep your camera ready—you may just witness your first smile or giggle! It might just be gas, but it's cute all the same.

▶ Other fun developments may include turning his head side to side, moving fists toward his face, visual tracking at close range, and even turning his head toward familiar voices and/or sounds.

NOT-TO-MISS APPOINTMENTS

▶ 3- to 5-day appointment

▶ 1-week appointment (if underweight)

▶ 2-week appointment

VACCINATION NOTE

Vaccination schedules are available from your pediatrician. You are the biggest advocate for your child. Don't be afraid to discuss this schedule and, if you have concerns, inquire about an alternative schedule, even if it's just to spread them out. Vaccines do come with risks, although the benefits tend to greatly outweigh them. Spreading the vaccines out a bit more means more trips to the doctor, but if your child has a reaction to one, it will be easier to know which was the cause.

Goals

STAFF MEETING

Get through the first week. This week is about survival, so lower your expectations right now. Eat standing up by the counter, no judgment allowed. We had *lots* of pizza during that first week, and many times we didn't even want to heat it up. You don't have to be on top of things—just focus on family. Most importantly, *accept help* in whatever form it's offered. And never forget you have a teammate—look out for each other when you can, and lean on each other when you have to.

HEALTH & WELLNESS

Get baby insured. You generally have 30 days after birth to add the baby to your health insurance, and this should be retroactive. Research the deadlines for your individual plan.
Watch the stump. When the umbilical cord is cut between baby and Mom, it's normally clamped with a plastic clip that resembles a mini potato chip clip, which is usually removed before leaving the hospital. It will take several days for the stump to dry out and fall off. My advice would be to avoid being nonchalant and oblivious; otherwise you may turn around and witness your Boston terrier gnawing on it after it fell off onto the floor. True story.
Defend from the touch. As a general rule, limit strangers touching the baby. If family and friends want to interact, please make sure that they wash their hands thoroughly. Your baby doesn't have the immune system to combat outside germs just

yet, and you are their only defense. Don't get crazy and ask people to shower, but good handwashing and common sense (don't kiss my kid!) goes far.

Know your upchucks. Spit-up is usually white with a tiny amount of what looks like curdled milk. If it's anything else or if you're in doubt, call your physician immediately.

Take time to interact. Your newborn is a sponge for input: Spending time talking, playing, and interacting with them is of paramount importance. It helps her push forward developmentally, and these are moments you'll never get back.

CRUISE DIRECTOR

Get outside. It's important for your well-being to leave the house. During my first few months at home with our first newborn, I was afraid to take her anywhere. I was nervous about how I would handle myself in public (not really knowing what I was doing), but more so about being able to negotiate strangers wanting to interact with her—plus the germs. Have a plan (keep baby tight to your body in a carrier or covered in a car seat/stroller), and you'll be fine.

SELF-CARE

Get some rest. Mommy is still in the recovery process, and you may also be emotionally spent. You'll hear it from a million different angles—sleep when the baby sleeps. It might be tough to catch ZZZs on command, but try your best—if you can't function properly, you can't be the best parent.

MR. FIX IT

Set up for success. Assess what you can do to make your home baby-friendly (noise-blocking gadgets or fans, extra pillows on the couch, strategic water bottle placed where Mom nurses [it's thirsty work!]).

DADDY DOULA

Be a diet detective. If your nursing baby is having digestive distress, gentle reminders to Mom about eliminating culprits such as milk products, caffeine, onions, and cabbage may help baby feel better and fart less.

BROWNIE POINTS

Label the goods. If your partner is producing enough breast milk to pump and freeze, step up and offer to catalog and label these bags. I kept the breast milk arranged in the freezer from oldest to newest. When Mom wasn't around, I warmed the first one up and loaded it into the bottle.

BONDING TIME

Start reading. It's never too early to start reading to your little ones. Start with picture books that have built-in sensory tools. There are a ton of books out there that help enhance and encourage the sense of sight, hearing, touch, and perhaps even smell.

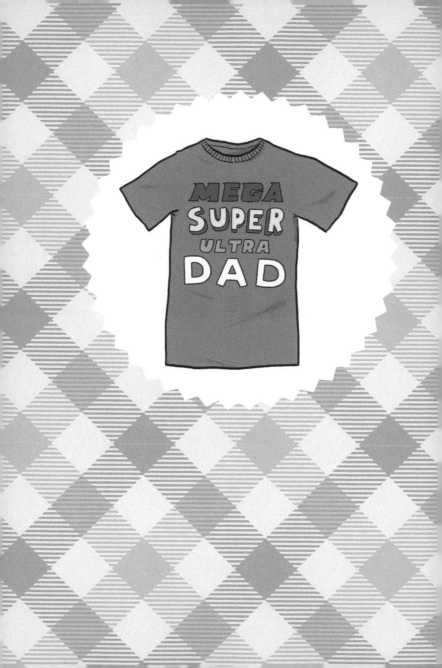

MONTH 2

AVERAGE SIZE	WEIGHT COMPARISON
10 pounds	Bowling ball, holiday ham

You've got a few weeks under your belt. But after the fanfare, people have gone back to their lives. If you were lucky enough to have them around, your parents and in-laws are long gone, and now you're an accomplished robot, a baby-handling machine. Shit is beginning to become utterly real.

With our first, Ava, my wife and I had all kinds of intentions of splitting up the nightly duties. The reality is, if Mom is breastfeeding, she's going to be up nursing. My wife would nurse, then wake me up, hand the baby to me to burp, change her diaper, and re-swaddle so she could go back to bed.

We really did that whole tag team thing. This works great, too, if you're bottle-feeding—you just each take a feeding straight through, and then at least you can get a few consecutive hours of sleep.

While most sources will suggest that new parents get the recommended 8 hours of sleep a night, more realistic numbers and recent studies show that you'll get, on average, around 4 hours and 44 minutes of sleep a night if you're lucky. Time to keep the cold brew ready.

Your baby will continue to find comfort in your touch, your snuggling, being close to your skin, and in most cases, Mom's breasts.

MOM STATS

▶ Mom is going through a hormonal shift. It's been natural to see her happy one minute and tearful or overwhelmed the next. This usually only lasts a few days and should have leveled out at this point. If it hasn't, talk with your partner and/or perhaps suggest that she speak with her physician about getting more support with this issue.

▶ If Mom had a C-section, she still shouldn't be lifting anything too heavy. She also may have a 6-week checkup scheduled with her OB/GYN.

BABY STATS

▶ Your baby is continuing to get stronger and show basic motor skills, including holding his head steady while being held upright, straightening his legs, and trying to kick.

▶ Your baby might begin to show excitement, happiness, and/or contentment.

▶ Your baby's grip is becoming stronger, and she's becoming aware of her fingers.

▶ Sight and hearing are becoming the leaders among sensory development—baby will begin to recognize parents' faces and react to big movements and colors with high contrast. Baby will also show emotion or reaction toward bigger noises directed at him.

▶ Keep looking for that smile—sometimes babies will respond with a smile to a parent's smile.

▶ Baby is reassured by parents' touch.

▶ You'll most likely begin to hear cooing and other sounds.

▶ Baby should be nursing 8 to 12 times over a 24-hour period, pulling down between 12 to 36 ounces of milk.

▶ Baby is sleeping between 14 to 18 hours a day, hopefully between 8 and 9 hours a night and 7 to 9 hours a day with three to five naps.

NOT-TO-MISS APPOINTMENTS

▶ Mom's 6-week postpartum appointment

   ▶ *OB/GYN will ask about any potential PPD (postpartum depression) concerns.*

▶ Baby's 2-month pediatric appointment

   ▶ *Ask what milestones to be watching for.*

   ▶ *Bring your list of questions, and remember, no question is too outrageous.*

   ▶ *Refer to your schedule of immunizations so you know in advance what vaccines are coming up.*

Goals

TAG TEAM

Stay the course together. Remember to have each other's back on a daily basis. Meeting challenges is something that is better done together than alone.

Find your groove. At this point, if you haven't found your tag team rhythm yet, it makes sense to pursue it. Sorting out responsibilities and deciding who handles what for work and home is of paramount importance for peace of mind and peace of home.

Hone your de-escalation skills. There's a fine line between soothing your baby using traditional methods and getting lazy and giving her to Mom to nurse. Make your best effort to exhaust the other reasons baby might be in distress (see How to Read Baby's Cues page 11 for a refresher).

HEALTH & WELLNESS

Watch for the ball drop. You'll want to keep an eye on baby boy's testicles as they continue to develop. It's normal for boys' balls to take several weeks, months, or even years to fully descend—but if they don't descend by 6 months old, it's important to get treatment. Make your pediatrician aware at each visit.

Care for the circumcision. If you chose to have your baby circumcised, as the circumcision continues to heal, you can ask the doctor if it looks okay and what things to watch for, such as penile adhesion (see page 19). Do your best to gently clean the area with a warm, damp cloth to remove any fecal particles or dirt.

BONDING TIME

Ease into sexy time. Most physicians will recommend waiting about 6 weeks before you begin to think about "extra-curricular activities." Be open and honest with your partner—there's no sense in rushing something that her body may not be ready for. Hormonal shifts and nursing could also play into your partner's excitement for or hesitation to having sex. Find other ways to be intimate—you can cuddle together and even resurrect the fun old pastime of "making out" if you feel up to it.

Keep talking. Yes, talk to your partner, but also give play-by-plays when talking to baby. When you're carrying them around, talk through what you're doing as you go about your day—babies soak it up.

Plan something for two. You and your partner could use a couple of hours out to remind you that you are still people, not just your baby's round-the-clock waitstaff. Is there someone you trust to care for your baby for a few hours? Maybe on a night when your favorite band is in town? Make a plan, man. Shed those too-short shorts and New Balances, and go have some different kinds of fun.

SELF-CARE

Exercise your body. It's extremely easy to become overwhelmed with the end of pregnancy and first few months at home. Sympathy weight is a real thing, and if you've had to extend your waistline by a belt loop or two, it's normal, but you'd better think about reversing the trend! Finding an hour to sweat helps not only your midsection, but your mind as well.

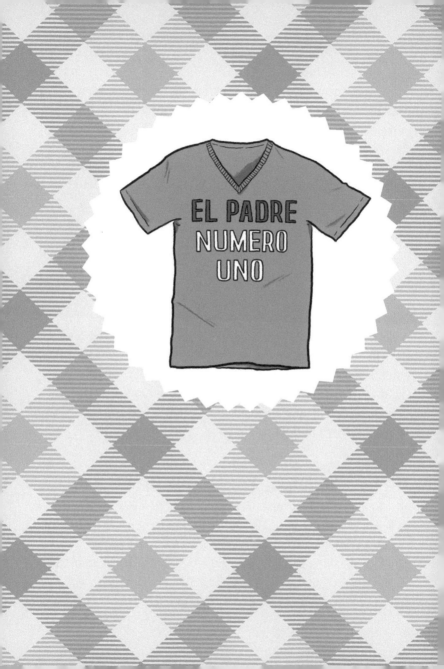

MONTH 3

AVERAGE SIZE	WEIGHT COMPARISON
13 pounds	Watermelon, an adult Maltese

If you're lucky, you and your partner have a system in place. But babies are unpredictable, so you're already starting from a position in which the unexpected will likely occur. Flexibility is key.

My hope is that your baby is gaining weight, eating regularly, and with any luck, you're seeing fewer bowel movements. You can start counting on naps. I remember how I would fantasize about naptime—I had grand plans of cleaning and paying bills. More often than not, I found myself reheating leftover dinner, turning the video monitor volume on high, and closing my own eyes. Which is sometimes the right answer.

This will be a big month if Mom is headed back to her job. This may be a really tough separation for her. Even if she is excited by the prospect of going back, it is still likely to be a very emotional day, week, and month. She may also be trying to get back to her pre-baby weight or having to adjust her wardrobe for an occupational setting. Maybe you're interviewing a nanny, babysitter, or daycare facility. Get in there. Offer a hand (or two), research, meet potential help, take some tours, and give input. Support one another.

MOM STATS

▶ Mom may be going back to work this month—issues to resolve may include childcare plans, transportation arrangements, pumping options, milk storage, and separation anxiety.

▶ Mom may be trying to lose some of the extra pregnancy weight—positive comments from a partner can go a long way!

▶ Mom's hormones are still adjusting. Continue to stay alert for signs of postpartum depression (page 7). Stave off feelings of isolation by getting out into the fresh air and socializing with others.

BABY STATS

▶ Baby may be having fewer bowel movements, which is okay if she is gaining weight and eating.

▶ Be vigilant against diaper rash (see page 65). Acidic poop and even dampness can aggravate baby's bottom and cause blisters.

▶ Baby should gain between 1 pound and 1¾ pounds this month, and lengthen by about ½ inch.

▶ Baby should be drinking 4 to 6 ounces at every meal, totaling 24 to 36 ounces per 24-hour period.

▶ Baby should be taking three to four naps a day and sleeping 15 to 17 hours a day.

- ► Motor skill development includes opening and closing hands, playing with hands, and bringing hands to her mouth, holding things, and swiping at dangling objects.
- ► Hand-eye coordination begins, and baby makes eye contact.
- ► Baby is getting stronger, perhaps raising his head and chest while lying on his belly, or holding his head steady while sitting in your lap.
- ► Baby is learning to self-entertain, and using expanding communication skills to express emotions.
- ► Baby may experience her first sleep regression. This is when the bedtime routine comes in handy.

NOT-TO-MISS APPOINTMENTS

- ► 3-month appointment
  - ► *Bring your list of questions and ask what milestones to watch for.*
  - ► *Know what vaccines to anticipate, if any.*

Goals

PLAN AHEAD

Plan for the sitter. If you don't already have one, make a babysitter checklist.

Start documenting. Still have that baby book sitting on the coffee table? Take a few minutes to jot a quick "funny" before you forget it. If the book isn't handy when something good happens, write it on a scrap of paper—you can transfer it to the book later (or just build a collection of scrap-paper stories). Remember that when all is said and done, you'll be left with the memories. Make sure you've got them stored somewhere.

STAFF MEETING

Plan Mom's return to work. Mom returning to work may feel like it's throwing a wrench in the system you were close to perfecting. Talk it through and revise that schedule.

HEALTH & WELLNESS

Know when to walk away. *Never* ever shake a baby in frustration. Aside from the obvious inhumanity of the act, it can cause severe damage to his developing systems or even worse, death. If you find yourself at a breaking point, hand baby off or walk away and take some deep breaths.

BROWNIE POINTS

Take the night shift. Offer to take some nighttime feedings so Mom can sleep through the night.

SELF-CARE

Find your tribe. Reach out to other new parents and find a new parents' playgroup or hangout. No one will be more understanding of where you're at mentally and physically than a handful of trusted peers.

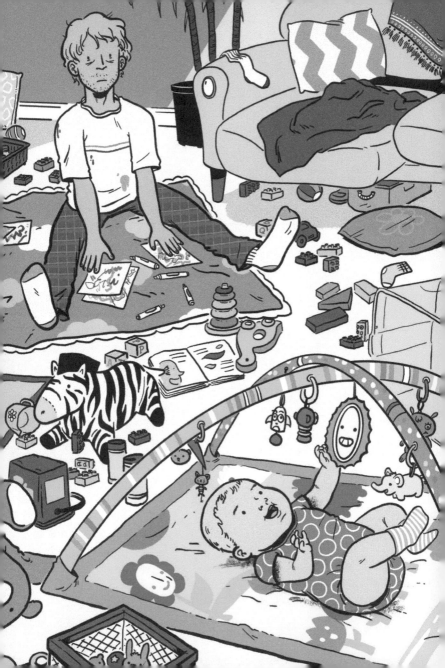

CHAPTER TWO

4 TO 6 MONTHS

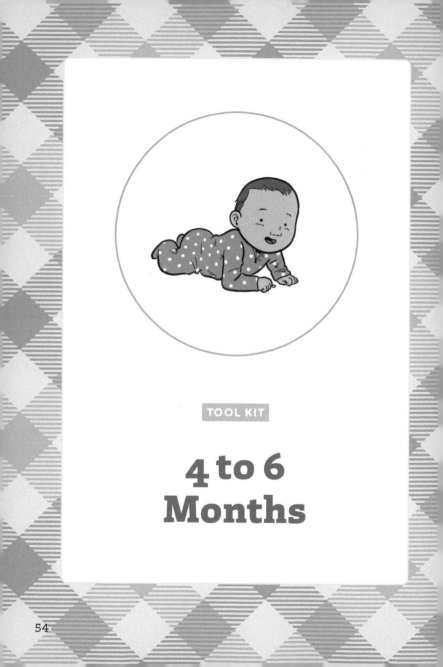

TOOL KIT

4 to 6 Months

4 TO 6 MONTH CHECKLIST

HOME

☐ Babyproof all accessible outlets with protective covers.

☐ Install baby locks on cabinets.

☐ Move chemicals to higher ground, out of baby's reach.

☐ Look at the world from a curious baby's vantage point. Get down low and look under furniture, coffee tables, and cushions. Notice all the fascinating things she will want to touch, knock over, and put in her mouth. Secure, move, or discard hazardous items or treasures.

BABY

MONTH 4

☐ Make sure baby only has access to safe items—she will begin putting everything in her mouth.

☐ Baby is becoming more mobile by the day. Make sure he's always well supervised and/or properly restrained to prevent falls.

MONTH 5

☐ Continually assess baby's surroundings for safety hazards; that is, anything baby can grab, eat, or knock over.

☐ Keep making space in your busy lives for quality time with baby. Her personality and capabilities are growing by leaps and bounds—don't miss a minute!

MONTH 6

☐ Find new games to play with your baby as he begins to sit. Keep baby surrounded by pillows so every landing is a soft one.

☐ Provide baby with lots of playthings in various shapes and textures.

☐ Experiment with sensory stimuli: splash water, blow bubbles, help her stand in the grass—it's all great exposure to her big new world.

☐ Kick-start baby's social circle with some playdates or story time at the library.

MOM

☐ Just like Dad, Mom will benefit from getting involved with other parents, whether she's back to work or not. Playgroups, playdates, story time, and Mommy and Me classes are a few of the ways Mom can connect with other moms and babies in real time. The folks you meet now will be running parallel to you for years to come, so keep in mind that from these kinds of groups, y'all may sprout some enduring friendships.

☐ Mom needs a date with you. By now I hope you have a trusted babysitter. Surprise Mom with a night out on the town.

☐ Check in with Mom about issues with breastfeeding or pumping.

☐ Be open and talk about sex and intimacy. She may also have some anxiety about her new mom bod.

MEDICAL APPOINTMENTS

☐ Time for your baby's 4-month and 6-month pediatrician checkups.

☐ Both of these checkups may include immunizations.

☐ Bring your list of questions for the doctor.

☐ Note baby's developmental strides—the doctor can confirm that baby's on track.

EVENTS

☐ Half-birthday: Half a year is something to celebrate. Even if it's just the three of you, make baby a crown and sing to him over a bowl of baby oatmeal.

Tips and Tutorials

Eat

HOW TO INTRODUCE SOLIDS

Most pediatricians won't recommend starting the baby on solid foods until around 6 months old, but if baby sits up well without support and you feel like he is ready, you can get started. One of the first things recommended is to start baby on an oatmeal or rice baby cereal. This is a low-allergen, bland food to start with. (Some people start their babies on fruit and then find that their baby has no interest in the blander foods.)

DO YOUR HOMEWORK. Look for an organic, whole-grain cereal fortified with iron, which helps the developing body and brain.

START WITH A RUNNY MIX. You'll want to mix a little cereal with water, formula, or breast milk (that's what we did) to achieve a runny consistency. Food can be room temperature or even a little cooler.

PREP AND SERVE. With a bib on baby and a soft cloth to spare, you can begin feeding. Make sure baby is fully upright. Place a minuscule amount of food on a baby spoon, and bring it to baby's mouth. If baby is as ready as you think she is, she'll open her mouth and accept the food that you smear into her mouth. This may take several attempts.

SAVOR THE EXPERIENCE. The first few meals are more about introduction than anything else—this won't replace their bottles quite yet! They will, as they saying goes, get more food on them than in them. But as long as they accept the spoon, continue feeding a bit at a time. When baby clamps her lips shut or turns away from the spoon, she's telling you "enough."

GO SLOW. Introduce just one new food each week, so you can see how he responds and pinpoint exactly where any allergies or issues may be coming from.

TAKE BABY STEPS. Once you've fed baby, say, oatmeal, for a week, you can move on to another food.

MIX 'N' MATCH. You can combine two previously introduced ingredients (for example, rice and pears) with your liquid, and serve them as a blend.

PERSIST. Sometimes it will take multiple attempts for baby to decide whether she loves or hates something. Her palate will change, and she'll suddenly get sick of something she loved. Just keep reintroducing foods every so often.

LIQUIDS

▶ Milk (formula or breast)

▶ Water

GRAINS

▶ Barley

▶ Oatmeal

▶ Rice

VEGETABLES

▶ Butternut squash

▶ Green beans

▶ Sweet potatoes

FRUIT

▶ Avocados

▶ Bananas

HOW TO MOVE BEYOND BASICS

Barring any contradictory advice from your pediatrician, you can begin introducing other foods. A few tips on this:

▸ Work your way up with textures. Start with runny foods and mixtures, and then work up to thicker mixtures as baby shows the ability to manage them. Make sure baby is able to mash foods to a consistency he can swallow. Of course, harder foods (like meat) need to wait until teeth arrive.

▸ When introducing eggs, make sure they're fully cooked.

▸ Make certain that all juices, milk, cheese, and dairy served are pasteurized. These should never be raw, as raw versions present the opportunity for bacterial infection.

▸ Do not feed a baby honey until after the age of 12 months. Bacteria found in honey can make a baby very sick (botulism).

▸ As she starts adjusting to food purées, she may like good yogurt frozen in tubes (skip the junk-laden Go-Gurt; go organic with this stuff) as an amazing treat. We buy Stonyfield Organic Yogurt Tubes, slice them in half, and freeze them (you can also cut them after they're frozen)—it's an awesome, healthy treat for baby that will do double duty in healing aching gums.

▸ Know that this does not have to mean the end of nursing. My wife breastfed each of our children until about age 2—they ate solid foods and she nursed them intermittently through-out the morning and evening.

HOW TO SPOT FOOD ALLERGIES

As you start introducing solid foods, certain allergies may rear their heads. Here are some things to know and tips.

KNOW THE BIGGEST FOOD OFFENDERS. The big eight allergens are milk, eggs, tree nuts, peanuts, soy, fish, shellfish, and wheat.

KNOW YOUR FAMILY HISTORY. Talk to your immediate family. If you don't have a significant family history of allergies, your pediatrician will likely give you the all clear to try anything (aside from honey).

INTRODUCE ONE FOOD AT A TIME. This way you will know what causes a reaction.

PAY ATTENTION. Most food allergy reactions occur within an hour of the food being eaten. A baby can have an immediate and scary reaction to a food (wheezing, difficulty breathing, swelling, severe vomiting, or diarrhea), in which case you'll call 911. Signs of allergy can include:

- ▶ Hives, welts, rash, or eczema on face, body, or diaper area
- ▶ Swelling of face, lips, or tongue
- ▶ Vomiting and/or diarrhea
- ▶ Coughing, wheezing, or difficulty breathing
- ▶ Loss of consciousness

FIND A GOOD ALLERGIST. If you suspect your baby has an allergy, make an appointment with an allergist. They will pinpoint the culprit and find a solution.

Soothe

HOW TO SOOTHE ACHING GUMS

Is your baby completely obsessed with his mouth? Drooling like a faucet and cannot keep his hands out of his mouth? Sounds like his chompers are getting ready to come in. You can help by providing your little one with tools to feel more comfortable.

▶ Rub your baby's gums with your clean finger.

▶ Offer a cool frozen washcloth or chilled (not frozen) teething ring.

▶ With your constant supervision, offer a cold hard food (like a carrot or bagel) to chew on. Be watchful, and take the food away if small pieces break off.

▶ Serve frozen tubes of yogurt, halved.

▶ Dose out some infant pain relief medicine.

HOW TO IDENTIFY AND TREAT FOR ALLERGIES

Your baby may develop a rash or get itchy, and you don't know where it's coming from. And not every allergy is a food allergy. Environmental allergies and adverse reactions to certain products are very common, especially with products that come into contact with baby's sensitive skin. Some tips include:

CHECK YOUR CLEANERS. If you're cuddling with your baby, wrapping her in swaddle blankets, or letting her lay on your bed for wind-down time, you'll want to think about the detergents you're using to clean these items, as well as any products you might be using on your face or skin—these things may not agree with supersensitive baby skin. You and your partner will come to find out in good time if your child seems bothered by scents and detergents. One of our children has more sensitive skin, like his old man, but the others never seemed to have any issues. All babies are different.

BE WARY OF ESSENTIAL OILS. There are a few places where the natural parenting community and good old-fashioned Western medicine tend to overlap, but often overlooked is the use of essential oils on or around newborns. Their skin is thinner and they can absorb dangerous amounts. Ask your pediatrician for suggestions if you're a fan of essential oils. Some essential oils are safe in certain applications, while others may not be. Play it safe and do your homework, then make sure all oils are included in your safety sweeps and placed out of reach.

BE A SMART SHOPPER. If you're like me, you tend to help by sharing the supermarket responsibilities. It's important to check the ingredients on anything that you're putting on your baby, whether it is shampoo, soap, lotion, or diaper cream. Check reviews online, and if your little one begins to develop a rash, discontinue use of the items that touched that area until you've figured out the culprit. The easiest way to know if a product is healthy is that it should have an ingredient list you can actually pronounce.

BE MINDFUL OF RASHES. With the onset of solid foods can come some diaper rashes. These rashes can indicate an allergy, which can become quite severe if not addressed. Consult an allergist, who can help you determine what food(s) might be causing this reaction. Change diapers as soon as they are wet or soiled. Use a clear barrier cream for protection, and for an active rash, use a thick cream with zinc oxide.

Sleep

HOW TO TRANSITION TO BABY'S OWN ROOM

You may be ready to reclaim your bedroom as your own. Here's how to make the transition as smooth as possible.

SET THE BEDROOM TONE. Establish the new bedroom as a place where quiet things happen. Avoid rowdy playtime in here—otherwise baby will associate the space with fun. Begin spending your quiet wind-down time in the new room. Sit and read books. Listen to soft music. Keep the lighting low.

HONOR THE ROUTINE. It doesn't matter the time of day that you're putting your kid down—think about the wind-down. This is the routine that tells baby "Full disclosure: bedtime is coming." Think about turning down the TV, turning down the blinds, and getting him into a darker, cooler, and quieter setting.

GET COZY. You can put her over your shoulder and walk with rhythm, or give her a warm bath and read a story. The object is to make her drowsy.

PUT DROWSY BABY TO BED. Some babies like to nurse to sleep. The experts will tell you this isn't a great idea because they fall asleep with milk in their mouth, which isn't good for their teeth, and they may not learn to self-soothe themselves to sleep. Ideally, you'll want to place a drowsy baby in bed and let him fall asleep on his own.

BE PATIENT. If baby wakes up after only a few minutes into a nap or nighttime slumber, let her try to fall back asleep, even if she fusses a little. It may take some patience to get her back to sleep. Rinse and repeat. Many people might tell you to let them "cry it out." My wife and I are not and never were fans of this method of parenting. That said, there is a difference between allowing a baby to fuss for a couple of minutes versus crying outright for half an hour, an hour, or, like our one foray into the CIO method, five hours.

A FINAL WORD OF ADVICE: All this said, you definitely don't want your baby to only be able to sleep in one type of environment or setting. Don't you want to go on vacation one day? Babies that are able to sleep through noise or can sleep in places other than their crib or car seat will be more flexible over time. And if you have a desire for your family to grow further, you'll consider this a win.

Learn and Play

HOW TO PLAY SENSORY GAMES

Your baby is a sponge, and playtime is of paramount importance to her development. Consider play her first job. You can help her along in this journey by inspiring play that engages all the senses.

And for all of your playtime, remember two things: get down there with baby and *you* are the best toy of all. You can play too, and baby will enjoy your company. Lay on the floor with your baby as he plays—no need for him to watch you sit on the sofa and smell your stinky feet from below. Engage baby with funny faces and copycat games. Let him explore your face and hands. Sing and dance together. Be the inventor of great activities that will deepen your relationship and help baby grow.

Some great sensory games to kick things off include:

WATER PLAY. Bath time is fun, but baby can also enjoy water play while sitting in a high chair or on your lap, indoors or out. Fill a pan with even the smallest amount of water, and baby can splash to her heart's content. Use a cup to pour water over her hands, or fill a squirt gun and spray her hands. Float a rubber duck and let her grab the moving target as it floats around. As baby gets older, you can add sponges, funnels, and cups with various holes in them for her to explore. Constant supervision is critical, however, even with a small amount of water.

PEEK-A-BOO. "Where is Daddy? Here he is!" Peek-a-boo gets fun reactions from baby, but it also teaches object permanence—a.k.a., just because you can't see something doesn't mean it's not there. You can also play peek-a-boo with a toy by placing a cup or towel over it and then removing it to reveal the toy—"Where did the block go? There it is!"

PLAY WITH YOUR FOOD. Yes, you may spend the rest of his childhood telling them not to, but playing with food is actually a great way to introduce foods and make them more acceptable. It also teaches baby that mushy, messy things can be fun. Place a small amount of mashed carrots on his tray and let him finger paint to his heart's content.

SENSORY TOYS. Anything that makes noise, squeaks, or rattles when pressed or shaken is great. Play mats and play gyms with toys attached are another fantastic option. You can make your own, too. Drum loud with pots and spoons. Or, if Mom's sleeping in, use plastic containers for your Zeppelin tribute.

HOMEMADE SENSORY BAGS. Check out Pinterest for a universe of sensory, squishy bag ideas. You don't have to be Martha Stewart to figure these out. Fill a resealable bag with a few small toys, sequins, sand, pom-poms, beads—whatever doesn't have sharp edges—and then add some cheap hair gel to make the bag "mashable." You can also simply fill the bag with water beads (you can find these online). Press the air out, seal with colorful duct tape, and then tape it to the high chair tray or a mat on the floor. You will be as obsessed with this toy as baby is. Good thing, because constant supervision is required for this one—it contains choking hazards and things you don't want baby ingesting.

SENSORY JAR. Fill a plastic jar with beans, rice, and toys, seal it tightly (reinforce with duct tape), and then set baby loose to shake and roll it around. Again, make sure you're present whenever baby's playing with your homemade toys.

Clean

HOW TO CLIP BABY'S NAILS

What a sweet baby. But those little wolverine nails can become a menace to your face, Mom's boobs, and any sibling's flesh they come in contact with. Your baby is old enough that their nails have separated from the skin, but it's still a good idea to stick with the baby clipper (they usually have a magnifying glass on them) so you don't lop off an appendage. Hint: It's sometimes easier to do this when they're asleep.

1. **Pull back the skin.** Use your thumb to gently press their fingertip pad away from the nail.

2. **Follow the curve.** Clip along the curve of the nail.

3. **Go easy.** No need to cut too low.

4. **File the nail.** Finish off by sanding down the rough edges with an emery board.

If you are fraught with worry about this task, skip steps 1 through 3 and simply sand down the nails. It will take longer, but it is a very gentle way to get those nails shorter.

NATURAL CLEANING SUPPLIES

With your baby on the verge of crawling, she's going to be touching everything in sight. With touching comes putting those fingers and hands in her mouth. While we often consider germs and dirt, it's also worth thinking about the cleaning supplies you use to remedy this.

REVIEW YOUR CLEANING SUPPLIES. What are you cleaning your carpets and/or floors with? What about baseboards or banister rails? Cabinets? Read the labels, then . . .

SWITCH TO NATURAL CLEANERS. Look for cleaners that are biodegradable, plant-based, hypoallergenic, free of dyes or synthetic fragrance, nonflammable, and contain no chlorine, phosphate, petroleum, ammonia, acids, alkalized solvents, nitrates, or borates. Natural food stores often carry environmentally healthy cleaning supplies, but so do an increasing number of supermarkets.

Babyproof

HOW TO BABYPROOF YOUR HOME: PART ONE

With crawling on the horizon, you'll want to make your home safe with a thorough inspection. Use the following to effectively clear the decks.

GET DOWN ON ALL FOURS. Begin your journey throughout the house on the level of your infant. (This could be a more exciting experience after an adult beverage or two.) As you crawl around, look at the things that your baby could potentially put in his mouth—loose coins, batteries, water bottle caps, pills or vitamins, slime, LEGOs, magnets (especially the magnetic balls, which can find one another after ingestion, causing intestines to pinch together to create a serious medical crisis), paper clips, small pieces of plastic or trash, and balloons from your last birthday party.

DESIGNATE THE BABY ZONE. Even if you're a fan of attachment parenting, you will find that it's necessary to put baby down from time to time, and having one designated safe area in the home is paramount. With all of our kids, we've had an actual baby zone that included a softer rug or rubber play tiles laid down with a "baby play yard" or "baby jail" enclosing it. We put baby's toys in there, and anything is fair game.

PLUG THOSE ELECTRICAL OUTLETS. There's nothing like jamming a pinky into an A/C outlet and getting blown across the room. Rough times. Outlet covers are very cheap, and they are available almost anywhere from Amazon to the dollar store.

WATCH THE CORDS. A lot of companies have eliminated the hanging window cord from blinds; however, if they're still there, put a knot in that bad boy and get it up to the top of the window where only adults can reach it. There have been several cases of babies and small children getting tangled and strangled. Also be wary of cords that might lead to lamps and irons, or even the hanging plant whose living appendage has draped itself south. All of these things present a potential danger.

STRAP IT ON. This has a brand-new meaning. We're talking about heavy furniture and TVs. Even though baby won't be pulling up for a bit, while you're doing your inspection, take some time to look at pieces of furniture such as chests of drawers, televisions, etc. You can buy furniture straps that bolt into the wall from the back of the piece and will keep it from toppling over onto baby.

PREP FOR PETS. We all love our furry friends, but with a little one crawling around, you've got to think about pet food and water dishes, litter boxes, cords that lead to heat lamps, and fish tanks or terrariums that may not be anchored to the wall. I will tell you, almost all of our children have ingested dog or cat food. Baby number four is currently 11 months and has just eaten a few pieces of (clean) cat litter. It's generally not the end of the world. Poison Control will already be on your speed dial and they might even know your name—this is okay. This is what they're there for. Anytime you have a question, they know the answer.

INCLUDE TOYS IN YOUR INSPECTION. Soft and cuddly can also be dangerous. Your baby is now able to grasp toys, and while they're providing a sense of comfort and security, you'll want to watch out for anything that could be a potential choking hazard. Buttons, eyeballs, and noses could potentially come undone and end up in their mouths. If it can fit in the baby's mouth, it's too small. This includes parts—you may think that a baby can't swallow a Matchbox car, but those wheels? Choking hazards.

SET BABY'S BED RIGHT. Remember how you were so stoked to buy that 3-in-1 convertible bed for baby? Make sure that the mattress is dropped to the lowest setting, so that when they start pulling themselves up in the middle of the night, they won't accidentally fall over the edge.

Baby Gear

Must-Have

▶ **High chair:** Could you live without your kitchen table? Well, this is baby's table, but it also serves as a good place to play or just watch you grown-ups hustle around the kitchen.

▶ **Baby carrier:** If you want to accomplish anything or go anywhere a stroller doesn't fit, a baby carrier is a must.

▶ **Stroller:** You probably have one by now (please stop lugging baby in their car carrier—that's just masochistic), but if you have more than one child, strollers to accommodate young siblings, twins, triplets, and beyond are available and recommended.

Nice to Have

▶ **Nursery camera:** For me, this is a must-have, but it's a personal thing. And for heavy (parent) sleepers or the parent who may be on a different floor than their baby, the audio/video component gives you that extra layer of comfort. Many will allow you the ability to observe the camera, as it's live-streamed to your phone via an app. With these new technological advances also comes the risk of them being hacked. Consider a VPN (virtual private network) and heed other users' advice.

- **Sleep sack:** Around this age, we let go of the swaddle and adopted a zip-up sleep sack. Perfect for when baby comes out of the bath.

- **Booties, socks, or shoes:** Keeping feet warm is key. Shoes are really not meant for walking at this age, so keep them lightweight, breathable, and comfortable. We always kept our babies in socks until around 10 months or later. Companies like Trumpette make cool baby socks that look like shoes.

- **Toys:** As mentioned, playing is baby's job. It will help him develop in every way. Anything that provides visual interest or makes noise or music is great. Surround your child with a variety of toys. When purchasing toys, use reputable companies, read reviews, make sure they're age appropriate, and play with it yourself to ensure that it's safe. All that said, don't disregard online yard sale groups or consignment shops for toys—some of the best stuff can be found there for cheap.

- **Old remotes or flip phones:** You may think this is a joke, but it's not. If my wife and I don't sell our old cell phones or home phones, we've always pitched them into a bin for the kids to play with. The buttons seem to be an endless source of fun and interest.

- **Baby swing:** We were gifted one of these with our first and it became a landmark piece in our living room, lasting us through all four babies' first 6 months of life.

- ▶ **Door jumpers:** This was also a key item when I was looking to accomplish anything in our common areas. They're inexpensive and fun and make it easy to contain baby.

- ▶ **Food purée machine:** Fun story about the Magic Bullet. My wife worked with Heidi Klum on a reality show, and she and her then-husband, Seal, gifted us one for Ava as we returned home. It's empowering to know that you control what goes into baby's body. To this day, we still make morning protein smoothies with it and it has survived the test of time.

Pass

- ▶ **Walkers:** Most, if not all have been removed from the market. Walkers are not recommended by the AAP (American Academy of Pediatrics) due to many kids pulling things down on their heads.

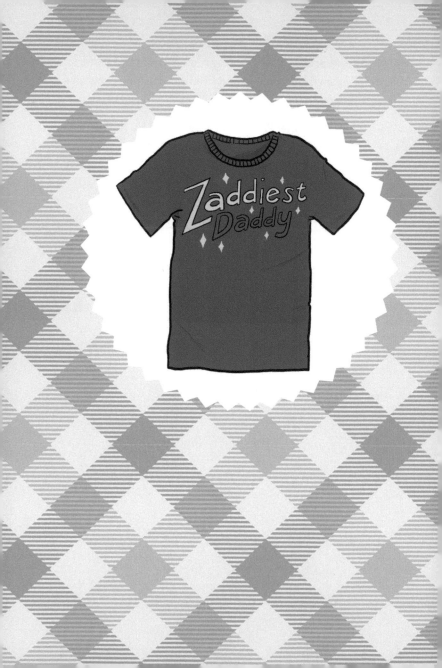

MONTH 4

AVERAGE SIZE	WEIGHT COMPARISON
15 pounds	Medium bag of dog food, a nice northern pike

You've been indoctrinated; you're a survivor.

The first 3 months as a new father are extremely tough. It definitely wasn't easy for me to make the transition—even as the older brother of three boys, I had never had anyone fully reliant upon me.

As an adult, I had mostly lived a decidedly single, self-centered existence. Getting engaged and married wet my feet in terms of shouldering the responsibility of another human being, but becoming a father flipped my world upside down.

You'll probably agree that those first 3 months are draining for both parents. But hopefully, you're now feeling more confident. With any luck, your baby has settled in. You've (hopefully) established an eating and sleeping schedule that allows you to find a few moments to connect with your partner.

However, just when you thought you had it all figured out, you might be facing one of the most challenging assignments. My wife describes this period as the "day after Christmas"—everyone has gotten to see the present (the baby), the initial excitement has worn off, and you're tired and cranky from too much hot cocoa and partying through the night. You're in love with the gift, but reality has set in, and the truth is *this shit is hard*.

The good news in all the sleep-deprived chaos: Whether you know it or not, you are getting better at this.

MOM STATS

▶ If Mom is still able to breastfeed, congratulations to her! This process takes a lot out of her both mentally and physically—baby is literally sucking the calories, vitamins, and minerals from Mom's body.

▶ If baby begins rejecting the breast, Mom will want to pay close attention to what she might be eating that's disagreeing with baby. Spicy foods or strong flavors may not fly, so start with simple fixes like cutting down on these to get clued into baby's resistance.

▶ My wife breastfed all four of our kids, but let it be said: the only wrong way to feed a baby is to not feed them at all. Breast, pumping breast milk, donor breast milk, formula, whatever floats your boat—as long as baby isn't losing weight, you're all good.

▶ Mommy may have used up her combination of paid/unpaid leave and may be looking at going back to work. This can cause stress with separation, scheduling care, and establishing eating, feeding, and/or pumping schedules.

▶ Postpartum depression can take months to surface. Big things to look out for are low moods that last for longer than a week, crying a lot, lack of appetite and/or libido, and feelings of inadequacy or rejection.

▶ Postpartum depression can occur in Mom or even Dad— this is different from baby blues (see page 7) and should be addressed immediately with your family doctor.

BABY STATS

▶ Your baby will typically gain between ¾ and 1½ pounds.

▶ They will grow probably close to ½ inch in length *and* head circumference.

▶ Baby has been sleeping more soundly, between 14 and 16 hours in a 24-hour period. But just when you've got the sleep schedule dialed in, you're about to embark on the exhausting 4-month sleep regression. This is when your baby all of a sudden goes back to a more newborn-style sleep pattern, waking very frequently at night. Although there are temporary regressions at 8, 11, 18 months, and 2 years old, the 4-month sleep regression is a permanent change to your baby's sleep cycle.

▶ Most night sleep is occurring in 6- to 8-hour increments.

▶ Expect two to three daytime naps, roughly 1½ to 2 hours each.

▶ Baby is nursing six to eight times a day. Overnight feedings are becoming less frequent. If feeding on formula, that frequency could change to four to six times a day, with 5 to 7 ounces consumed at each session for a total of 24 to 32 ounces over 24 hours.

▶ Baby is likely beginning to suck on her fingers and hands.

▶ He will become fussy when forced to sit or ride in a car seat for extended periods of time.

▶ Keep an eye out for the mini-pushup. When baby is lying on his stomach, he will attempt to use his arms to push his upper torso into the air. It won't last long, but practice makes perfect.

▶ Rolling is something that can make a debut, so don't take the chance of leaving baby on the sofa or bed unattended.

▶ Strength and motor skills development continue as baby may:

 ▶ *Hold her head steady while sitting up.*

 ▶ *Hold a toy and shake it to hear sounds.*

 ▶ *Pick things up slowly and release them.*

▶ Sensory development strides may enable baby to:

 ▶ *Study and explore small items.*

 ▶ *Stare at things in the distance.*

 ▶ *React to sounds and possibly search for them.*

 ▶ *Laugh and giggle with individual interaction.*

NOT-TO-MISS APPOINTMENTS

▶ 4-month appointment: Compare stats from last appointment. Tell the doc what baby's doing and ask if you're on target developmentally. The pediatrician will be depending on your observations of these things, as your baby may not perform on command during the appointment. Suggested immunizations could include:

 ▶ *DTap (diphtheria, tetanus, and pertussis)*

 ▶ *Hib (Haemophilus influenzae type b)*

 ▶ *IPV (inactivated poliovirus)*

 ▶ *PCV (pneumococcal)*

 ▶ *RV (rotavirus)*

A NOTE ON INTIMACY

Let's talk about libido. In my experience, after having a child, nothing is the same for a while. My wife sometimes wasn't ready for sex for a couple of months, and that was okay with me. Her body had been through a lot and she was recovering, bonding with baby, and trying to find her way again in a new body she didn't necessarily recognize. I made sure she knew I found her incredibly, over-the-top sexy and attractive, but did not try to pressure her. I made sure to kiss and hug her, and to occasionally playfully pinch her tush. But even though I know my wife was grateful, I also know she experienced a difficult time—how do I put this delicately?—separating herself from her breasts. She says that as we got near the time when sex was going to naturally be back in the game plan, she began to pull away from me. She was uncomfortable with her breasts and the role they had always played in our sex life. She felt like they were, temporarily, there for the baby and therefore off-limits for me. She had a hard time "flipping the switch" between nursing our child and sexual intimacy, and I had to, and did, respect that. All this to say, take the time to talk with your partner about sex, and allow her to take the lead. Just like men don't always know how they're "supposed to feel," women have these moments of self-doubt as well.

Goals

HEALTH & WELLNESS

Create a veggie lover. Even if you don't love your veggies, baby may. Getting baby to eat fruits and vegetables in the coming months will be easier if a nursing mom incorporates a large amount of them into her diet. Many food flavors are passed on through amniotic fluid and breast milk. So eat a wide variety at meals—you too, Dad.

Treat a teether. If your baby is chewing on his fingers a ton, it may be a sign that a tooth is making its way to the surface. Baby can't yet grab a chilled teether from the refrigerator—it's up to you! Offer a chilled teething ring, for everyone's sanity. There are also teething mitts that you can Velcro onto your baby's fist like a mitten, but the top of the mitt is a teething pad. Babies this age don't have the dexterity to hold a teether, so this is a great idea to help teach baby to self-soothe.

TAG TEAM

Tag team diaper changes. With learning to roll comes a feisty baby who will generally not want to cooperate while you're changing her. When possible, work as a team and take turns holding legs and occupying her with songs or engaging her with conversation.

BONDING TIME

Wear your baby. Don't be afraid to go to your local retail or boutique store that focuses on baby gear. Try on a few different baby carriers. There was no way that I was getting anything done on a daily basis or on the weekends if I wasn't able to put my kid on my back, side, or chest. Just don't think you're going to operate the stove or deep fryer with them on up front.

Take a day trip. One of my favorite pictures is of me carrying my son Mason in an external backpack to the top of Stone Mountain in Georgia, and I keep it framed in my office. It's really easy to stay at home in your comfort zone, but stepping away and doing something adventurous makes for great memories.

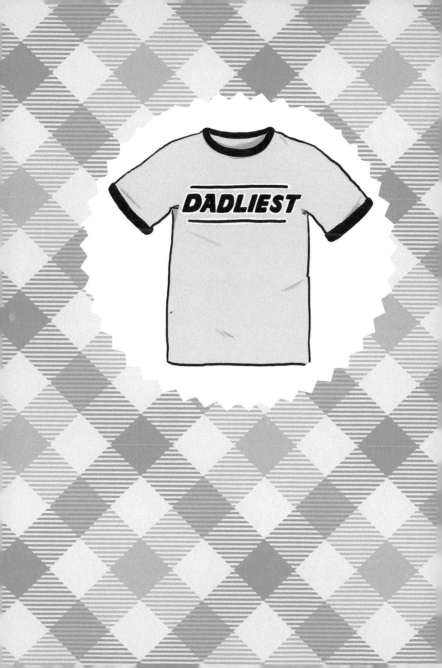

MONTH 5

AVERAGE SIZE	WEIGHT COMPARISON
15 to 16 pounds	19-inch flat-screen TV, sperm whale's brain, overweight cat

Welcome to Droolfest—you've got VIP, all-access passes for the entire show.

Your baby may be teething up a storm, with slobber pouring out. All four of our kids popped their first teeth around 6 months, and those few weeks leading up to it included many crying solos—pretty sure I even contributed to one or two duets out of complete frustration.

As we've touched on before, with kids, once you think you have their behavior patterns dialed in, developmental milestones will throw you a curveball. With each new phase generally comes new sleep patterns, changing eating habits, and moments of fussiness.

But that's just one side of it. On the bright, sunny side of all of this, your baby has had a fair amount of time to adjust to Mom, Dad, and family life. She is becoming more interactive and showing glimpses of emotion, desires, and true personality. Every sight and sound attracts her attention.

You'll also begin to notice your baby having increased control over his body. Fingers, toes, and everything he can get his hands on will start going into his mouth. And while that's simultaneously exciting and potentially disgusting, pretty soon you can begin to think about introducing his mouth to another thing—solid foods. This is huge!

MOM STATS

▶ Mom should be fully adjusted to the new normal of your family. If you still have PPD (postpartum depression) concerns, address them with her and help facilitate an appointment with her physician.

▶ If she's still breastfeeding, she may be considering how long to do so. Try to be a supportive listener and ask what you can do to help.

BABY STATS

▶ Baby will likely gain 1 to 1½ pounds.

▶ Baby will grow by about ½ inch in both length *and* head circumference.

▶ Baby is sleeping about 15 hours a day with 10 to 11 hours of sleep per night.

▶ Expect two to three daytime naps, each typically between 1½ and 2 hours.

▶ Your baby is still on a mostly liquid diet.

▶ Baby is feeding five to six times per day, consuming 24 to 36 ounces over a 24-hour period.

▶ Strengthwise, baby is rolling along, literally. Also, baby may be able to sit upright on her butt on the floor while balancing with hands at her sides. She may also be able to bear weight on her legs for a few seconds.

▶ From a motor-skills perspective, baby is now able to grasp toys, even with two hands, and is working hard to get toys that are out of reach. And almost everything is starting to go in his mouth.

▶ Sensory development means baby may be studying small objects for longer periods of time, quickly locating sources of sounds, and making expressions such as laughing, showing dislike, fussing, crying, or even pushing away. He also may begin to cry when interaction ends.

▶ Teething may start. Early signs are drooling, chewing on fingers and everything else, slobbering like a rain gutter, and a chin or face rash. Baby may even start pulling on ears—gums, ears, and cheeks share the same nerve. You may think they have an earache, and then all of a sudden you will see a white spot on their gums and boom—tooth! I've noticed that the hard part of teething is the cutting: once the sucker pops through, the fussiness tends to wane. Teething note: Lower central incisors generally appear between 6 and 10 months, lower lateral incisors between 10 and 16 months, upper central incisors between 8 and 12 months, and upper lateral incisors between 9 and 13 months.

  ▶ *Early teething cues can be obvious fussiness or even baby beginning to push his body up while on his belly.*

NOT-TO-MISS APPOINTMENTS

▶ Medical checkup for Mom and baby

Goals

PLAN AHEAD

Make a feeding plan. While most pediatricians won't recommend solids until baby is 6 months old, start reading up and talking about it.

CRUISE DIRECTOR

Carve out couple time. For the first few months, you and your partner may feel like ships passing in the night. You're likely working, trying to maintain a household and keep a little one alive and happy, all while balancing competing schedules. There isn't a whole lot of time alone. It's important to stay connected. In the early days, my wife and I would find time to connect early in the morning or late at night, generally while the baby was asleep. As you continue to build your squad, this becomes harder and harder to accomplish, but it's important to keep in mind. When your relationship is solid, the kids feel it.

HEALTH AND WELLNESS

Bring the outside in. Adding plants to the house is something we've consistently tried to do, as it is proven to improve the air quality inside the home. Bring home some flowers or a potted plant, which also scores you brownie points—double win.

Prioritize water quality. If you're formula feeding, you probably already know about the importance of spring water, or at the very least, highly filtered water. Our water supply contains a lot of heavy metals and even remnants of pharmaceuticals, so getting our house on a system for clean water was important and beneficial for everyone. We use a PUR filter on our kitchen sink, but there are a lot of other affordable options.

 BONDING TIME

Mix things up. It's very easy to lie there with baby resting on your chest and watch endless TV—and sometimes this is *exactly* what is needed. But if you're this far along in this book, I'm confident this is not your default dad position. I get it. It's easy to get in a rut and run the same plays over and over. Today, you should call an audible. Run a different route. Find another place to hang out. Come up with some new material. Let baby chill with you in a different position. Communicate in a different way. See what happens.

BROWNIE POINTS

Commit random acts of awesomeness. Baby is 5 months old, so you should be starting to catch your breath as routines develop. Just like with baby, don't let routines with your partner turn into ruts or complacency. Shake things up in a good way by complimenting and showing affection to your partner every day. Seek out thoughtful deeds, whether it is bringing home flowers, sending Mom out to spend an evening with friends, or finally tackling something on that honey-do list. And if all that is beyond your reach right now, even something as simple as leaving a Post-it note with a heart on her steering wheel can make a difference in how she approaches her day.

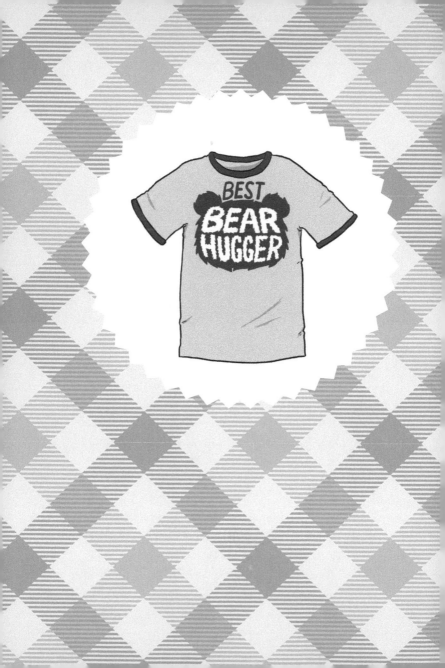

MONTH 6

You're about 6 months in and those teeth that were bugging your little one may have busted through! Keep an eye out; the lower central incisors generally pop first.

It's time to expand the culinary horizon and experiment with different foods. Sure, 85 percent of this will end up on your kitchen floor, with 65 percent of *that* stuck to the bottom of your feet, or smashed onto their hair, bib, or seat tray.

One thing I love about this phase is that everything they're seeing or doing is *new*. Watching your friends post their never-ending "baby's firsts" was annoying—but now you get it. Your little human is beginning to have more core control, his motor and sensory development is improving rapidly, and it's becoming a lot more fun to play with your baby.

You're approaching the official half-year mark, and my guess is that you're awakening and seeing how much more there is to life.

MOM STATS

▶ Mom may feel self-conscious or frustrated if she hasn't returned to her pre-pregnancy weight or shape. Chances are you haven't been able to shed that "sympathy weight" either. You *both* may be contending with stretch marks, changing of breasts, and continued hormonal shifts, but this stat isn't for you. Remind her she's beautiful.

▶ If Mom is nursing, she may be continuing full on or she may be weaning. If she's weaning, she can get pregnant. This is a good time to remember that the rhythm method may not be the best choice of birth control.

BABY STATS

▶ Expect 15 hours on average of sleep—10 or 11 at night and 3 to 4 hours of daytime naps between two or three naps.

▶ Based on your pediatrician's recommendation, your baby is clear to start eating solids.

▶ This is arguable, but breast milk may not be enough to provide the amount of protein, iron, zinc, and other vitamins that baby requires to develop. One of our babies didn't start solids until almost 10 months, and we just added a baby multivitamin drop to her morning routine.

▶ With solids being introduced, your baby's poops will change—say goodbye to that sweet-smelling Dijon. They'll become darker and eventually more composed.

▶ Baby is starting to sit up, maintain good head control, and roll over back to front and front to back.

► Teething is real—feel the gums for any new arrivals.

► Baby is using motor skills to pull or rake small objects toward herself on the floor, enlisting both hands to pick up objects or toys, and putting anything and everything into her mouth.

► Baby enjoys simple games and exploring his fingers, toes, legs, and ears.

► Baby may start expressing herself with vowels. Giggling and laughing is a daily occurrence.

NOT-TO-MISS APPOINTMENTS

► 6-month appointment: Compare stats from your 4-month appointment and bring a list of things baby is doing so you can confirm that everything is in line developmentally. Tell the doctor what your baby is doing so doc can confirm.

► Vaccines: Once again, the AAP will recommend that your baby receive the following, but the decision is solely yours as parents:

 ► *IPV (polio)*
 ► *PCV (pneumococcal)*
 ► *Hep B (hepatitis B)*
 ► *RV (rotavirus), depending on vaccine given*

Goals

STAFF MEETING

Take stock of your partnership. This 6-month milestone is a great time to look back together and ask "How'd we do? What worked? What didn't? How can we improve as parents? Are we taking care of each other and our relationship? Are there any stuck points or areas of concern?" A little brainstorming may reveal some telling truths and some agreeable solutions.

PLAN AHEAD

Explore food options. Starting baby on solid foods opens a whole new world of possibility. Explore brands and styles. Pouches are easy to take on the go, but they're not the most environmentally conscious choice. Consider making your own purées and freezing them. Or not.

Consider drafting a will. This is one thing that may be easily avoided, but you'll want your baby protected should something happen to you or your partner. It's an important, if uncomfortable, conversation to have.

CRUISE DIRECTOR

Offer opportunities for movement. Heavy or large motor skills take practice and a lot of it. Provide him with a lot of opportunities for sitting, crawling, and climbing. From sitting to lying on her stomach to lying on her back, let baby stretch her arms and legs. Pull her into sitting position, sitting in a tripod, sitting upright, standing on your lap or chest/stomach and bouncing, pulling to standing with your fingers.

Work fine motor skills. Practice dexterity by giving baby different things to hold, pick up, and grasp—I often let our baby crawl to me and drop things in her way for her to pick up. We play finger or hand games: Patty Cake, sooo big, and high fives are favorites. We also pick out physical attributes: pointing to our noses, eyes, ears, etc.

Play word games. Focus on single words with your baby and talk slowly. Repeating and asking them to do the same will eventually reap big rewards.

HEALTH AND WELLNESS

Help baby along with teething. You should routinely feel their gums. Signs of teething are drooling, irritability, crankiness, diarrhea, swollen gums, and chewing on fingers or solid objects. Help him feel comfortable by providing a chilled teething ring or those frozen yogurt tubes.

SELF-CARE

Assess your dadness. Use this month to reflect on the kind of father you are, and wanted to be, when you first thought about fatherhood. Are there any gaps? You may realize you're not as patient, social, or active in decision-making as you hoped you'd be. Maybe you'd hoped for more alone time with your partner. Use this month as a turning point—work toward being the dad you know you can be.

Evaluate your health. A lot has changed in the last 6 months. As you reflect, make sure that includes considerations for your physical and emotional well-being. If there's anything you need to do to step up your self-care, pursue it.

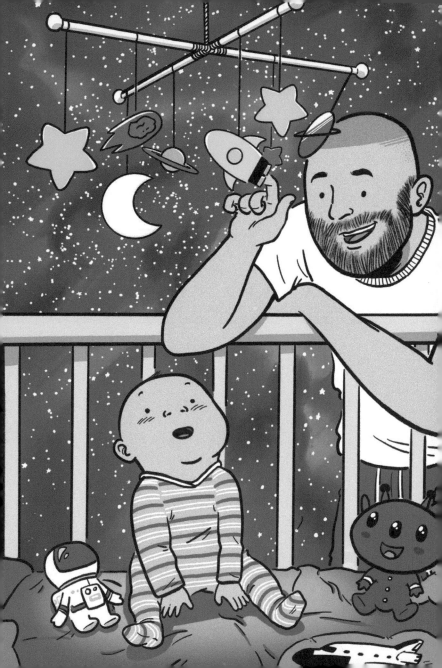

CHAPTER THREE

7 TO 9 MONTHS

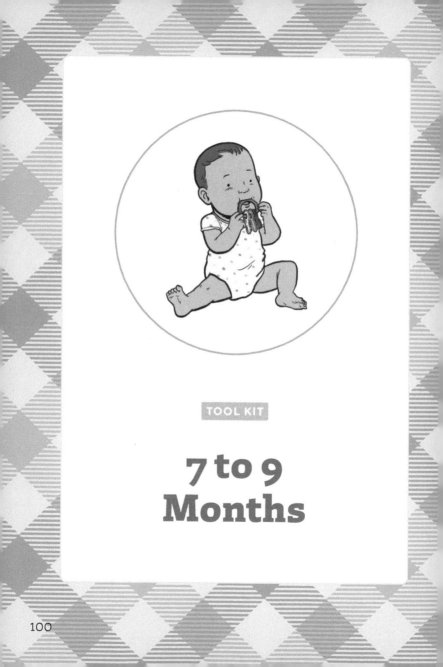

7 to 9 Months

7 TO 9 MONTH CHECKLIST

HOME

☐ If you haven't yet, lower the crib mattress. If your baby is sitting up, she's probably also on the brink of pulling herself into a standing position. It's time to search furiously for the crib manual and drop that baby mattress down to its lowest setting. If you don't get ahead of it, you run the risk of having your baby go butt over teakettle and end up hurt, or free outside the prison grounds, crawling to freedom elsewhere in your house.

☐ Continue vigilant sweeps of the home and floor for baby hazards. Keep in mind that he can reach farther than you think he can.

BABY

MONTH 7

☐ Expand baby's culinary horizons, one ingredient at a time.

☐ Begin finger foods (see page 104).

☐ Try taking baby out to dinner, if you haven't already.

☐ Help him with teething woes.

☐ Encourage baby's mobility, creativity, and curiosity through a wide variety of toys, games, songs, and stories.

MONTH 8

☐ Continue baby's bedtime ritual. He may experience another sleep regression, and that bedtime ritual will help wind his busy mind and body down.

☐ Provide lots of opportunity for movement, crawling, and play. If you don't let baby practice during the day, she will want to practice at night!

MONTH 9

☐ Offer safe, sturdy furniture for baby to pull himself up with. Move wobbly stuff to another room for now.

☐ Continue vigilant hazard sweeps. Keep in mind that baby can reach new heights and will continue to surprise you.

☐ Use a firm, gentle "no" when baby tests the limits.

MOM

☐ If Mom is still breastfeeding, she may be dealing with challenges such as pumping, clogged ducts, or weaning. She is also burning through a lot of calories, so she should replenish her own stocks by eating a wide variety of good foods.

MEDICAL APPOINTMENTS

☐ The next checkup may not be until baby is 9 months old, so in the meantime, don't hesitate to schedule an appointment or call the doc with any concerns you have.

Tips and Tutorials

Eat

HOW TO CREATE A SUPPLY OF BABY FOOD

Making your own baby food is easier than you think, and it
has many benefits, including being cheaper and healthier than
buying off the shelf. Here's how to get started.

1. **PREPARE YOUR FOOD.** Purée your foods using a food
   processor or by hand. Rather than using salt and sugar,
   you can season foods with herbs and spices like cinnamon, garlic, ginger, allspice, basil, mint, and more.

2. **STASH IT.** Prepared foods can be transferred to a covered
   ice cube tray, tiny freezer-safe containers, or reusable
   baggies labeled with food name and date.

3. **STOW IT.** Store food in the refrigerator for up to 4 days,
   or freeze for up to 3 months. Defrost in the refrigerator
   overnight, or use the defrost feature on the microwave.
   Always stir well and test food before feeding it to baby.

4. **OPTIMIZE LEFTOVERS.** Rather than toss dinner's leftovers
   or an overripe banana, purée them for future baby meals.

Once baby has gone through the single-ingredient purées and seems ready for the next step, it's time for finger foods. Baby will *love* the control he suddenly has over what food he's eating. And if you have a hungry Boston terrier, they'll love the scraps!

START SMALL. The key to finger foods is to start very small and soft. Try these winners:

- Small cooked pasta like ditalini
- Pancakes, cut into tiny bites
- Cereal circles
- Baby puffs
- Bits of crackers
- Tiny cubes of soft cheese or shredded cheese
- Scrambled eggs
- Cut-up fruit (avocado, banana, pear, peach, apricot, cantaloupe, kiwi, mango, honeydew, blueberries)
- Cooked, cut-up veggies (carrot, potato, and peas are good starters)
- Shredded chicken or fish fillet

WATCH CLOSELY. You will still want to supervise baby while he eats. Eating even just a tiny bite of cracker, if baby is stuffing his cheeks with 10 bites of cracker, this can cause a mushy choking hazard wad. Make sure baby is taking time to swallow before eating more, otherwise you can just start by putting out one or two bites at a time.

AVOID HARD, ROUND, OR STICKY FOODS. You may have grown up on hot dog "nickels," but we know now that rounds are perfect choking hazards. The same is true of foods like raw veggies, grapes, raisins, popcorn, and peanut butter.

STARTER FOODS	7 TO 9 MONTHS

LIQUIDS

▶ Milk (formula or breast)   ▶ Water

GRAINS

▶ Barley   ▶ Rice

▶ Oatmeal   ▶ Pasta

VEGETABLES

▶ Butternut squash   ▶ Carrots

▶ Green beans   ▶ Peas

▶ Sweet potatoes   ▶ Potatoes

FRUIT

▶ Apples   ▶ Cantaloupe

▶ Avocados   ▶ Honeydew

▶ Bananas   ▶ Kiwis

▶ Pears   ▶ Mangos

▶ Apricots   ▶ Peaches

▶ Blueberries

PROTEIN & DAIRY

▶ Cheese (small cubes)   ▶ Fish fillet (cut up)

▶ Chicken (shredded)   ▶ Tofu (small cubes)

▶ Eggs

SNACKS

▶ Crackers

Soothe

HOW TO MAINTAIN THAT LOVING FEELING

Now that baby's not a newborn, you may feel like things have sped up and you're not getting in the cuddle time you used to enjoy together. Fear not—baby still needs lots of love and reassurance. Here's how you can help:

RESCUE THE WEARY TRAVELER. As baby begins to gain the ability to venture away from you, your very presence is critical to his feelings of security. Baby may be crawling backward and have little ability to get back to you, or may just get tired, so if he starts to fuss, scoop him up and give him a big hug.

SOOTHE YOUR TEETHING LITTLE ONE. Teething can make for a fussy baby who just can't get comfortable. Cuddle in and rub those sore gums, will ya?

INSTILL A SENSE OF SECURITY. Some babies begin having separation anxiety at this age. You can help reassure baby that you are someone she can count on. Make goodbyes quick and upbeat. Try to leave when baby's happy, such as after a nap or feeding. Play peek-a-boo to help teach baby you're not really gone.

MASTER THE BEDTIME RITUAL. If you're not on it, get on it. The bedtime ritual is your time to simply be together on the coziest of levels, to read and chill and cuddle to your heart's content—and it can help you handle the next round of sleep regression (see page 108).

Sleep

HOW TO HANDLE SLEEP REGRESSION. Babies go through a sleep regression around 3 to 4 months, and then another one around 8 to 10 months. It's said to be caused by baby's brain development, and can cause disturbances in sleep patterns. He can't fall asleep. He's practicing his new skills. Or he's just got too much going on in his head. (Can't you relate?) The good news is that his normal sleep habits will resume once baby's gotten the hang of all these new skills. In the meantime:

- ▸ **Rock that routine.** Now is an important time to ensure a solid bedtime routine. The bath, the books, the dimmed lights—pull out all the stops to make sure baby knows it's bedtime.

- ▸ **Allow for good naps.** Baby actually needs more daytime sleep, not less, when nighttime sleep is compromised. An overtired baby has an even harder time staying asleep.

Learn and Play

HOW TO MAKE GAME-PLAYING FUN FOR YOU, TOO

Yes, babies love games like peek-a-boo, Patty Cake, the Itsy Bitsy Spider, sooo big, This Little Piggy, eyes-nose-mouth, stomach raspberries, etc. But when you just need to step up the entertainment value for yourself, here are a few ideas.

PLAY PRETEND. I was never a theater major and, though I coached stand-up comics, I never took the stage myself. However, I always had a flair for acting wild (with or without beverages) and there is no better audience than a baby—he won't judge you. Quite the opposite, in fact. So find your inner Mrs. Doubtfire and have some fun.

SHARE A LULLABY YOU CAN RELATE TO. Rockabye Baby! has put out more than 80 releases of lullabies inspired by songs from your favorite bands. This is a perfect way for you to enjoy your music with your little one without blowing out their eardrums quite yet.

Clean

HOW TO KICK OFF GOOD DENTAL HYGIENE

Tooth buds are beginning to appear, and you'd better be ready. Here are some tips to set up baby for good dental habits.

START IMMEDIATELY. As soon as the first tooth appears, you'll want to clean it after every meal. You can use a damp washcloth, gauze, finger, or toothbrush to clean the teeth and front of the tongue. If you use a toothbrush, use a very soft one designed for infants.

LIMIT TOOTHPASTE. Keep toothpaste to a mere "grain" of a baby-friendly brand.

Babyproof

HOW TO BABYPROOF YOUR HOME: PART TWO

With your little one becoming mobile, you'll need to further batten down the hatches for their safety and your sanity. Focus on the kitchen, bathroom, and nursery.

▸ Any cleaners at baby level are a *no*. Put them up!

▸ Install baby gates between rooms and at the tops and bottoms of stairs to reduce the risk of them falling down, reaching balconies, or leaning on banisters, poles, or railings.

- Secure heavy furniture like dressers, nightstands, or end tables. If he can use any part of these to pull himself up, his weight can pull everything down on top of him. Nightstands and end tables should also be cleared of any hazards.

- Cords for lamps, laptops, kitchen appliances, blow-dryers, hair straighteners, etc. need to put away or hidden to restrict access for little crawlers.

- Pick up a few dozen outlet protectors and plug up those power outlets. This is a great activity for older siblings—just make sure they don't miss any.

- Be wary of fireplaces, baseboard heaters, portable floor heaters, furnaces, and radiators. Restrict baby's access with portable gating.

- Houseplants are wonderful for the air, but can also pose a problem for kids who have no qualms about eating leaves and dirt, which can be poisonous.

- Make sure all doors are fixed with safety knobs (you know, the ones that we have trouble opening ourselves) and that there are locks or safety guards for windows above the ground floor.

- Speaking of knobs, you'll want to purchase and install some oven and stove childproof knob covers, especially if you have a gas system in the kitchen.

- In addition to cleaning products, cosmetics and hair care products should be moved up to higher ground. Look into a lock or guard to secure the toilet and vanity. And while you're babyproofing, find a better spot for the toilet brush. I cannot imagine a long enough baby bath after *that* interaction.

- Do a higher-level inspection on the tops of low-lying furniture like coffee tables, end tables, and nightstands for choking hazards, prescription bottles, glass objects, etc.

- Be sure you've covered:

    - Curtain/blind drawstrings

    - Pet food and water bowls

    - Pest traps

    - Prescription bottles

    - Glass objects

    - Exercise equipment with moving parts

Make Your Own Cleaner

We've discussed that with baby touching *everything*, the cleaners you use are as important to consider as the dirt you are cleaning up. Make your own healthy, safe, effective disinfectant cleaner:

1. Combine 4 cups of water with ¼ cup of vinegar and 1 tablespoon of baking soda.

2. Add about 12 drops of tea tree or lavender essential oil or the juice of half a lemon.

3. Use as a disinfectant to clean general areas like high chair tops, changing tables, cutting boards, sinks, toilets, etc. Shake before using to emulsify the ingredients.

Pediatric

How to Deal with Common Illnesses

Day care is a hotbed of fun, activity—and germs. Whether your baby is in day care or home with you, she is eventually going to get some germs that make her sick. Here are some common ailments, signs and symptoms, and treatments.

COLDS. Baby colds are challenging, because babies haven't figured out how to breathe through their mouth. Just imagine how hard it is to suck a bottle or breast with a clogged nose. But getting plenty of fluids is important when baby has a cold. Call the pediatrician for advice. Doc may recommend saline nose drops to thin the mucus and then to aspirate baby's nose with a bulb syringe. Use a cool mist humidifier. If baby has a fever, that is her body's way of fighting infection. Your pediatrician will be able to give you recommendations on how to bring the fever down.

RSV. Respiratory syncytial virus causes infections in the lungs and respiratory tract. While very common, in more serious cases, it can land your baby in the hospital. Signs of mild RSV include dry cough, low-grade fever, stuffy or runny nose, and sore throat. More severe signs can include wheezing, fever, severe cough, labored or shallow breathing, tiredness, decreased appetite, and irritability. If baby has difficulty breathing, looks like he is "pulling in" around his collarbone or rib cage when he breathes, or has a blue color to his lips, seek immediate medical attention—don't wait for the doctor. My wife and I just went through this with our youngest, Evelyn. It seems to always happen or become an overwhelming concern over the weekend, when your pediatrician is off living their own life. Use your gut in this situation. If you have to make a trip to the local children's hospital at 3 a.m., then that's what you need to do. Evie has been admitted twice, once for RSV and once for HMPV (human metapneumovirus), while I was writing this book. She was held in pediatric ICU for several days, and while that's emotionally conflicting, I always knew that that's exactly where she needed to be to get well.

EAR INFECTIONS. Baby's ear canal is not fully developed—it's short and wide, opening the door to infection. Ear infections may be accompanied by irritability, fever, and pain, which can be identified by baby pulling on her ear or increased crying when lying down. Antibiotics are usually prescribed; offer baby a fever and pain reliever, and try holding a warm compress over the infected ear. Some natural healing websites offer insight on safe essential oils you can use.

COXSACKIEVIRUS. This common virus can cause a fever (and only a fever, in half of the cases). It can also cause hand, foot, and mouth disease, which causes painful rashes or blisters in the mouth (making swallowing painful) and on hands and feet, as well as conjunctivitis (pink eye). Viruses are not treatable with antibiotics—talk to the doctor, who will determine the course of treatment based on the symptoms.

CROUP. This barking cough can alarm parents with its sound. With our third baby, we called the paramedics at 1 a.m. because it sounded so scary. It's caused by an infection that obstructs the airway, which causes the barking sound. Yes, call the doctor, but in the meantime, sitting with baby in a steam-filled room can provide relief. Run a hot shower and bring baby into the bathroom, close the door, and let the baby breathe the steam.

CONJUNCTIVITIS. Otherwise known as pink eye, this eye infection causes redness, discharge, excessive tearing, and itchiness in one or both eyes. It's very contagious but is easily treated with antibiotic eye drops or ointment.

A NOTE ON FEVER/PAIN MEDS: Ibuprofen is an effective pain and fever reducer. There are studies that show that while acetaminophen reduces fever, it is not as effective for pain. Also, infant acetaminophen is very potent, and can cause liver damage if given in child doses. Always follow the directions on the label.

A NOTE ON COLD MEDICATIONS: Cold and cough medications should not be given to children under the age of 2.

Baby Gear

▸ **Tippee cup:** A cup with a weighted bottom will not only stay on the tray of the high chair, but also hopefully teach your little one to keep the cup in front of him, rather than on the floor. Oh yeah, it also teaches him how to use a cup.

▸ **Hook-in seat:** This type of seat comes in handy on a daily basis at the kitchen table, but also when you're able to take your baby out to eat with you on that 5 p.m. early bird reservation. Just be wary about the types of tables that you hook this to—make sure the table is sturdy enough to handle the weight of your baby.

▸ **Sling/baby carrier:** Have I mentioned this? Doesn't matter, I have to say it again: I wouldn't have gotten anything done *ever* if I wasn't able to strap this kid to my chest.

▸ **Toothbrush:** Get a soft-bristle toothbrush to use with baby toothpaste.

Nice to Have

▸ **Wagon:** There's nothing better than getting your baby out of the stroller and into a different mode of transportation. We added the canopy option, as well as the bag that hangs onto the back of the tail seat—the canopy is great to protect against sun and the elements, while the bag allows you to store drinks, snacks, a blanket, etc.

▸ **Grocery cart liner:** This thing came in handy more than I expected. Not only does it slip over the front seat of the shopping cart, it also doubles as a liner for most high chairs in restaurants—those things are the worst germ factories ever.

▸ **Portable pop-up crib/Pack 'n Play:** We've used one or two of these over the years—they come in handy for playdates, visiting at a relative's house, or a hotel stay. If you visit Grandma a lot, keep one all set up over there. I promise she won't mind!

▸ **Play yard:** Also known as a "baby jail" in our house, you can find pop-out versions and collapsible versions with detachable/attachable segments. This can come in handy when paired with an umbrella for a day at the beach or park.

- **Action and reaction toys:** Encouraging exploration and curiosity is paramount to good development. A few options to keep in mind:

  - Different-sized rings

  - Activity cubes

  - Balls that roll

  - Toys that encourage standing

  - Colorful board books

  - Sensory board books (the *That's Not My* . . . book series by Usborne Publishing is a great option)

  - Teething toys that vibrate

  - Toys that mimic your phone or tablet

  - Musical toys

PARENTING HACK TIP

If you're the one buying the musical toys, there's nothing wrong with taking a few minutes to explore these sounds. What if you were kidnapped and blindfolded, tied to a chair, and forced to listen to this for hours on end? Would you be able to endure the mental anguish that often rides alongside these toys? Elmo is pretty fun, until he's not. "Baby Shark" is cute, until you pull over at a rest stop, barricade yourself in the restroom, and refuse to come out. Choose wisely, New Dad!

- **External back carrier:** If your baby is able to fully support his head and has demonstrated strong neck muscles, you can carry him for a hike or a walk through the park or even have the carrier pull double duty for a quick turn around the grocery store.

Pass

- **Fresh food feeder:** The mesh or silicone personal feeders were never a huge hit in our household. They seemed to cause more frustration with the babies than good.

- **Teething tablets:** We tried these with our first and second, but let them go with the next two. Overall, the product didn't provide the relief that was promised.

- **Slip-proof baby kneepads:** Seriously?

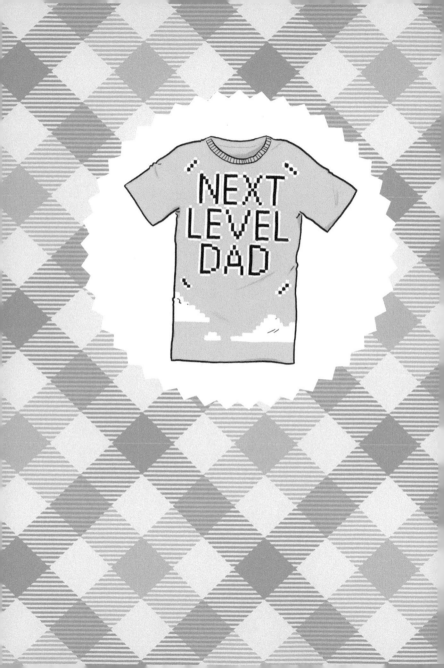

MONTH 7

AVERAGE SIZE	WEIGHT COMPARISON
16 to 17 pounds	28 rolls of toilet paper

My friends always said these few months exist to make you realize how easy a newborn is. I'm sort of kidding, but not really.

The reality is that as hard as the first 6 months are, your baby's been in what's commonly called the "potted plant phase," meaning you put your baby somewhere and he stays put. This quarter of the year sees that "potted plant" analogy go right out the window, which means many things, but mostly that you have to be on your game at all times. The good news is that this stage also brings with it fun milestones and physical advancements.

These few months bring more exploration of solid foods. When we first started having kids, pediatricians shied away from recommending more allergy-inducing foods (such as dairy and strawberries) until after 1 year old. Now, with our fourth kid, our pediatrician has changed their tune and said that it's imperative that babies try *everything* (except honey) by the time they hit 1 year old. Apparently, the response to the research telling parents to hold nuts until later was causing the rate of allergies to actually increase. Your doctor may say differently. Regardless, the traditional foray into solid foods is organic baby cereal. We only served this once a day, in the evening, because it is a meal that (selfishly) helped baby to stay fuller longer and thus sleep more soundly during the night. Hope that helps!

MOM STATS

▶ If Mom is still breastfeeding, challenges may include pumping, clogged ducts, or weaning.

BABY STATS

▶ Physical growth isn't that substantial.

▶ Baby should sleep between 9 and 11 hours each night.

▶ Baby will likely sleep 3 to 4 hours during the day, split up into morning and afternoon naps.

▶ Teething continues, as teeth may begin to pop through.

▶ Most of baby's nutrients are still derived from nursing or formula via bottle, even if she's eating solids.

▶ Baby will feed 4 to 6 times a day, drinking between 24 and 30 ounces per day.

▶ Once baby starts eating solid food, the amount of total daily intake may range from 3 to 9 tablespoons.

▶ Baby is responding to the word "no."

▶ Baby is responding to things like laughter, blowing in his face, blowing bubbles, and stomach raspberries.

▶ Separation anxiety is a real thing. Baby may begin crying as soon as he is put down and might be extremely attached to his primary caregiver. He is able to tell the difference between strangers and family.

▶ Baby should be able to hold herself up, sit unassisted, scoot, crab-walk, and/or crawl. Baby looks for dropped toys, and is able to reach and pick up favorite toys.

▶ Baby may be working on holding and drinking from a cup and/or eating from a spoon.

▶ Baby is developing his own personality and imitating words and speech patterns.

NOT-TO-MISS APPOINTMENTS

▶ No scheduled pediatric appointments

Goals

SELF-CARE

Unleash the beast. Join a gym. Maybe even consider a family membership and one that has day care. Our gym in Virginia has an amazing childcare component for all ages: crawling areas for toddlers all the way up to video games for those on the verge of becoming tweens. They'll watch our baby for up to two hours, which gives us some time to build some muscle and blow off some steam (or perhaps inhale steam in the sauna, like my wife enjoys doing).

MR. FIX-IT

Make a calendar. Since baby's arrived, how many special days have you forgotten about? Hopefully nothing serious, but if you've gotten burned by the missed-anniversary silent treatment, take time this month to jot down key dates and appointments on paper or in Google Calendar. And if you're having trouble remembering to pick up the dry cleaning, it's time to start keeping a to-do list. Leave a pad on your nightstand or add to your notes app, because you'll remember most of it at 3 a.m.

HEALTH AND WELLNESS

Learn first aid. Take a CPR class and learn the Heimlich maneuver. Knowing what to do if your baby chokes or stops breathing is one of the greatest insurance policies you can take out as a parent, and it will give you tremendous peace of mind. If Grandma and your favorite babysitter are up for it, consider treating them to the class as well.

CRUISE DIRECTOR

Go out to eat. It's inevitable. At some point, you'll need to bring this baby out into the world—to a restaurant. I hope you've done it before now, but if not, grab that hook-in seat, a bib, a few toys, some puffs or precut finger foods, and light up the town.

 STAFF MEETING

Put away the guns. If you own firearms, you're more than likely responsible and practicing your own safety protocols. If not, becoming a parent is the perfect time to tighten your personal gun laws. Guns should be unloaded with the safety on. If not already in a gun safe, at the very least, they should be put up in a restricted area—perhaps a finger lock or lockbox is something to consider. As an additional point, as your children get older and start having playdates at other people's homes, you should *always* feel as though you can ask this question: "Do you have unlocked guns in your home?"

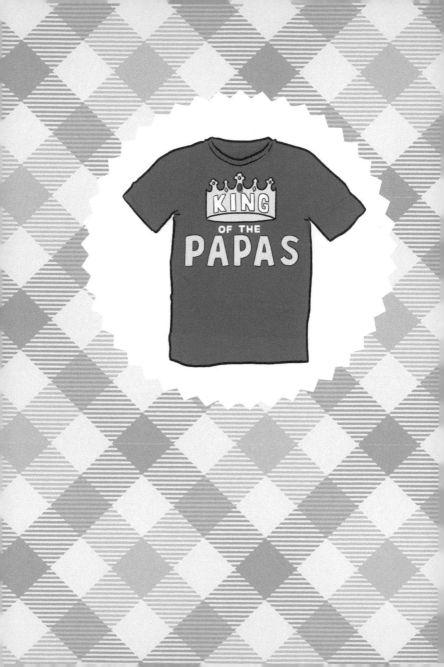

MONTH 8

AVERAGE SIZE	WEIGHT COMPARISON
17 to 18 pounds	Mini-keg, 77 blueberry muffins

One of the best parts of this phase is that your baby starts having incredible reactions to everything—your face, familiar pets, fun songs ("Baby Shark" has given me several migraines; the upside is that Evelyn calms instantly when she hears it). Your baby may be scared easily, giggle incessantly, and when someone raises their voice (in a family our size, it's destined to occur several times a day), you can see her eyebrows raise, and she pays close attention to the noise.

Prior to having kids, I didn't realize that these little guys were going to be fixtures in our bedroom for a *long* time. That's not for everyone, but it has really worked for us.

For the first half of the year, we used the co-sleeper, but around this time our baby began sleeping curled up next to my wife, who slept facing into the center of the bed with one boob out all night. Evelyn had commandeered that nipple; she could find it anytime (without night vision goggles). It became easy for my wife to nurse on demand and thus, not be tired for work the next day. Plus, I think the added cuddle time she got somehow made leaving for work in the mornings more bearable. Remember, this is what worked for us. I make no excuses for a deviation from what the experts will tell you. Again, I'm no Dr. Spock—just an experienced dad.

MOM STATS

▶ If Mom is still breastfeeding, challenges may include pumping, rejection, clogged ducts, or weaning.

BABY STATS

▶ Baby is likely getting 9 to 11 hours of sleep each night.

▶ Expect 3 to 4 hours of sleep during the day over two naps: morning and afternoon.

▶ Baby will be drinking between 24 and 30 ounces; however, with solids, these quantities will decrease.

▶ Baby will eat 4 to 9 tablespoons of cereal, fruit, and vegetables spread out over two to three meals.

▶ Baby may gain as little as a pound this month.

▶ Baby could grow as little as ⅜ inch; head circumference doesn't change much.

▶ Baby has almost mastered crawling and pulling up on things.

▶ Baby is laughing, exploring, discovering, and learning.

▶ Baby is experimenting with vowels in making sounds— A, E, I, O, U!

▶ Baby might bang blocks together or on things, toss or hold and drop balls, and put things inside of other things.

▶ Self-exploration is happening: baby will be pulling on ears and nose and discover genitals.

▶ Conceptualization of object permanence is setting in—for instance, when Mom or Dad leaves the room, baby still knows they exist and potentially calls for them.

▶ Baby is sitting up straight (unaided) and observing everything around him.

▶ Attaching motions with meanings of words; for example, waving and saying "goodbye."

▶ Baby is possibly stringing together combinations of words; saying "Mama" or "Dada."

▶ Thinking processes becoming more complex.

NOT-TO-MISS APPOINTMENTS

▶ No scheduled pediatric appointments

Goals

Find tag team opportunities. You're probably settled into a pretty predictable groove, but there's always room for improvement. Look for something your partner could use a break from and snap up that chore they hate, like washing the dinner dishes or folding laundry. Take something off your partner's plate, and say, "Tag, I'm it." For extra brownie points, make it your new duty for the long term.

Do a daily sweep. At the end of every day, I do a quick vacuum or sweep to clean up old baby puffs, shrapnel from the older kids, wayward pet hair tumbleweeds, and so on. Crawling babies will put *anything and everything* in their mouths. The five-second rule no longer applies. Work together and see who notices what.

CRUISE DIRECTOR

Make a baby date. Are you being social? Have you met any other parents? Can you count the times you've taken baby out without Mom on one hand? If you are hanging your head in shame here, make it a plan to take your baby out. Tell Mom to put her feet up—you're going on a baby date. Walk around the block, go to the playground or library together, or wander the aisles of your local hardware store.

Go somewhere fun. Babies this age really start to soak up their surroundings. This month, start trying out some completely new experiences as a family. Perhaps it's the zoo or a carnival. Maybe you're brave enough to handle a music festival or the state fair. Take lots of pictures and wash baby's hands well after touching the petting zoo animals.

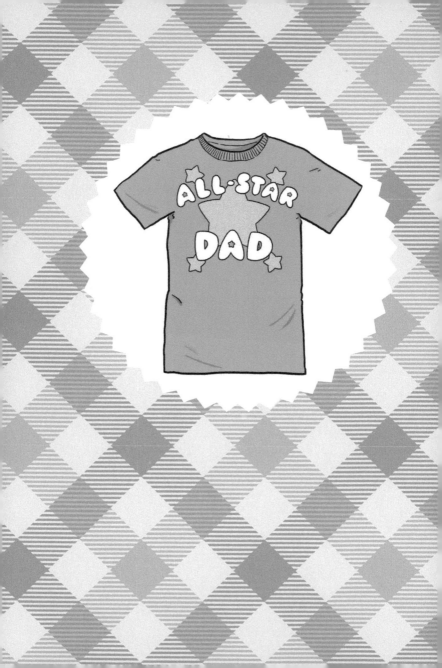

MONTH 9

AVERAGE SIZE	WEIGHT COMPARISON
18 pounds	Thanksgiving turkey big enough to feed a good crowd

Last month, I offered up a reference to the "Baby Shark" song that serves as ground zero for my migraines. That song may feel particularly relevant these days with those new teeth popping through, especially for Mom. You'd think those little Chiclets were laser-cut blades for cutting open bank vaults. I've watched my wife scream in agony after our little one almost took off her entire left nipple, slicing it to bleed. Be a team player—get some rubber chew toys, quick.

This first-year stage also marked the hardest of childproofing times for us. Once your little rascal starts cruising and eventually begins walking, it's time to lock it down. Remember—*everything* must go up. Your best bet is to again crawl around your home on all fours—pretend to be a baby, now having access to a completely new set of fishing grounds. It's amazing how much stuff we have at shin level. Don't get overwhelmed—make a list and lock down one room at a time. You can always use gates or a baby jail to keep them contained.

This is also a great month to ask your pediatrician those Facebook-inappropriate questions like "Is it normal that sometimes my kid looks at me cross-eyed?" Or "My baby ate dry dog food. Now what?"

MOM STATS

▶ If Mom is still breastfeeding, challenges may include pumping, rejection due to lower supply, clogged ducts, or weaning.

BABY STATS

▶ Baby is sleeping an average of 10 to 12 hours a night.

▶ Expect two naps between 1½ and 2 hours long.

▶ Feeding via breast milk: nursing between four and five times a day, drinking between 24 and 30 ounces per day, with quantities slowly decreasing as baby eats more solid foods.

▶ Feeding via formula: baby is downing between three and four bottles a day with between 7 to 8 ounces of formula for a total of 21 to 32 ounces, with quantities slowly decreasing as baby eats more solid foods.

▶ Baby is eating 4 to 9 tablespoons of cereal, fruits, and vegetables spread out over two to three meals.

▶ Finger foods are in full swing, and baby may eat between 1 and 6 tablespoons of meat, chicken, fish, tofu, eggs, or beans per day. Note: Baby can't digest fully—often, stuff looks the same coming out as it does going in.

▶ Baby may like playing with toys with buttons, levers, and dials.

▶ Crawling is almost perfected, but now baby is working on pulling himself up and standing with support.

▶ Baby is now making intentional actions and noises with toys for attention and is able to point, clap, and wave arms to get attention.

▶ Baby is babbling, pushing syllables together, and attempting to verbalize familiar words.

▶ Baby is beginning to test her limits and is very attentive when looking at parents and their reactions.

▶ Baby is giving limited time to strangers and focusing mostly on Mom, Dad, and siblings.

NOT-TO-MISS APPOINTMENTS

▶ 9-month appointment: Compare stats from your 6-month appointment and consult your pediatrician to make sure everything is within the acceptable developmental range. A few things your doctor may be looking for:

  ▶ *Baby's weight, length, and head circumference*

  ▶ *Screening test for early identification of developmental delays*

  ▶ *Information on eating habits and changes in peeing and pooping*

  ▶ *Daily sleep habits*

  ▶ *Is baby saying "Mama" or "Dada"; does she understand "no?"*

  ▶ *Is he sitting without support? Pulling himself up to stand?*

  ▶ *Is she walking with the aid of furniture?*

  ▶ *Is he responding to games like peek-a-boo?*

▶ Vaccines

  ▶ *The AAP will recommend that your baby receive a flu vaccine.*

  ▶ *If you're working on an alternative schedule, use this visit to catch up with a missing vaccine.*

Goals

MR. FIX-IT

Find your hammer. It may have been a while since you've tackled any home projects, but surely there's work to be done. This month, see what you can do to shorten that honey-do list. Hang that picture, spackle that hole. You have to keep your handy skills fresh; before you know it, your baby will be asking for a tree house.

Continue babyproofing vigilance. Work together or take turns scanning your home for new hazards. Always be watchful—learn to scan whenever you put baby down. Take five minutes as often as possible—ideally, daily—to go through the rooms of your home with a critical eye. And work as a team—you will each spot different things. And extend this same vigilance when you go to someone else's home—different homes, different hazards.

STAFF MEETING

Update important digits. Take a few minutes to research your local emergency numbers. These will come in handy for that babysitter you might eventually trust, as well as in the event that something happens on your watch. Include poison control, pediatrician, any specialists you may have, the emergency room, and nearby neighbors that can help in a jam. You need to have a village, even if you don't have family close by; rather, *especially* if you don't have family close by. In our neighborhood, our neighbors are our village, and we all look out for one another's kids.

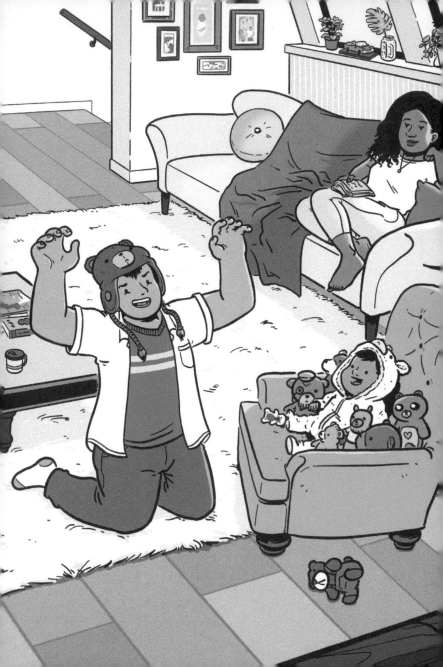

CHAPTER FOUR

10 TO 12 MONTHS

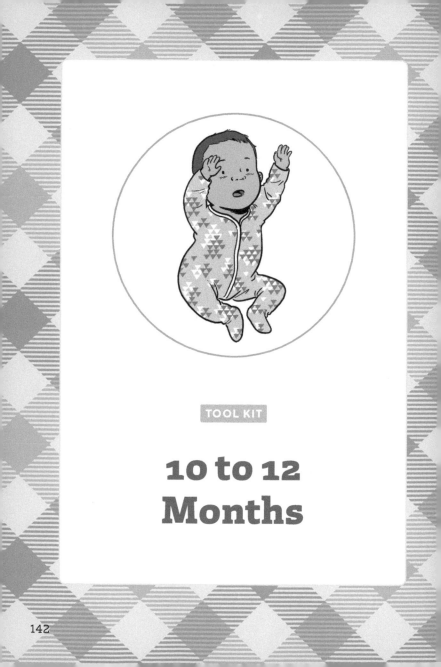

TOOL KIT

10 to 12 Months

10 TO 12 MONTH CHECKLIST

HOME

☐ Begin adding higher areas to your babyproofing inspections. Baby may be able to pull herself up, so it's all fair game—tabletops, sofa and chair cushions, toilet bowls, beds—the list goes on. Make sure the toilet is locked or secured and surfaces are clear of hazards.

☐ Baby can pull down lamps, chairs, stools, and the stove or dishwasher door. Always supervise baby when he's roaming, and provide sturdy, safe furniture to support him as he moves around.

☐ Make sure gates are sturdy and well secured and that baby's weight won't knock over a stair-top gate. Close doors to rooms that are off-limits, including bathrooms, basement, garage, and older siblings' rooms.

BABY

MONTH 10

☐ Nearly 75 percent of babies are sleeping through the night at month 10. If you're in the other 25 percent, you may want to consider sleep training, although I'm not personally a fan.

☐ If baby starts testing limits, know that he might surprise you with how he can get into trouble. Keep him safe and respond to "tests" gently but firmly.

MONTH 11

- ☐ Expose baby to different kinds of food. Know that it can take 8 to 12 tries for her to be able to either enjoy it or show lack of interest. If she doesn't like it, try reintroducing it later.

- ☐ Introduce baby to different textures. Their sense of touch is important to develop, and it helps make them more well-rounded and accepting of varying textures.

- ☐ Read to them every day. Point at things, identify them, and repeat yourself.

- ☐ You can begin to reinforce good behaviors and offer praise.

- ☐ You can correct inappropriate behavior by adjusting your tone. No need to yell—let baby learn by your tone, not your volume. As they get older, you can enlist the crazy side-eye, too (also known as "the look").

MONTH 12

- ☐ Let baby help parents while getting dressed, such as putting arms or legs where they need to go.

- ☐ It's okay to make the transition to regular cow's milk; however, don't use low-fat milk until after his second birthday.

- ☐ Be watchful and firm. At this age, she is testing limits—for instance, going up the stairs, seeing how much food she can throw on the floor before you correct her, getting into things previously unexplored. Say "no" gently but firmly, and move her out of the situation.

- ☐ Remember all the big events that this month brings—time to get baby's 1-year portrait done and plan a birthday party!

Tips and Tutorials

Eat

HOW TO ENCOURAGE A GOOD EATER

Do you eat to live or live to eat? Your baby is likely to emulate your habits, so make them good ones. Here are some tips for shaping your baby into the best kind of eater.

MAKE MEALTIME TOGETHER TIME. As often as you can, sit down with your baby when she eats. Eat alongside her. She'll watch you and learn from you (so use your napkin!). This also introduces the ceremony of mealtime, and in particular, dinner-time, which as your baby gets older, can be the perfect family time for catching up each day.

ENCOURAGE, DON'T FORCE. If you make a big fuss over what baby's choosing to eat, it's likely to create an issue. Just let him eat, and if he doesn't like something after a couple of tries, let it go. You can reintroduce it another time.

EAT THE RAINBOW. A colorful plate is so much more fun than one made of just one hue, and colors equal variety when it comes to nutrition, too. So mix up your food choices with reds, yellows, blues, and of course, greens.

FEAR NOT THE GREEN. Don't let any bias you might have affect your child's view on greens. It's all in the preparation. Serving chopped fresh broccoli sautéed with a little butter will likely give you a veggie eater for life. Roasting is another gateway to loving vegetables like Brussels sprouts, broccoli, and butternut squash—it brings out their sweetness. Just make sure they're cut up small enough to manage.

DON'T OVERSALT. It's a good habit to avoid adding additional salt to baby's food. They get enough with what it already contains, and you don't want him to get hooked on it. Explore other foods, spices, and herbs to flavor food—consider cinnamon, nutmeg, ginger, garlic, basil, dill, oregano, chives, pepper, curry powder, Parmesan or other cheeses, oils, vinegar, and lemon juice. Just remember that honey is off-limits for the first year.

GO WHOLE. Of course, baby would love to score some canned soup and a Twinkie. But processed foods tend to contain loads of salt and sugar, as well as other ingredients that set your baby's palate on hyperdrive and aren't conducive to your growing baby's health. The more whole foods you can offer, the better. Try your hand at homemade soup, mac 'n' cheese, pasta sauce, or hummus—they're all better choices than their prepackaged counterparts and honestly fairly easy.

GET CREATIVE. The more options you provide, the more variety baby will be exposed to, and the more adventurous an eater he is likely to become. My wife and I have a food blog called Think Outside the Lunchbox, which started out as simple toddler and preschool lunch ideas and has slowly expanded. Get beyond peas and carrots and consider foods such as these:

- ▶ **Dairy:** Cottage cheese, yogurt, cheese—American, cheddar, or something mild like Monterey Jack or Parmesan

- ▶ **Fruits:** Papaya, watermelon, plum, and strawberry

- ▶ **Vegetables:** Steamed cauliflower or asparagus, diced sweet potato or baked eggplant, cut-up roasted green beans or butternut squash

- ▶ **Grain:** Quinoa, couscous, brown rice, and amaranth

LIQUIDS

▶ Milk (formula or breast) ▶ Water

GRAINS

▶ Barley ▶ Amaranth

▶ Oatmeal ▶ Brown rice

▶ Pasta ▶ Couscous

▶ Rice ▶ Quinoa

VEGETABLES

▶ Butternut squash ▶ Sweet potatoes

▶ Carrots ▶ Asparagus (cut up)

▶ Green beans ▶ Cauliflower

▶ Peas ▶ Eggplant

▶ Potatoes

FRUIT

▶ Apples ▶ Mangos

▶ Apricots ▶ Peaches

▶ Avocados ▶ Pears

▶ Bananas ▶ Papayas

▶ Blueberries ▶ Plums

▶ Cantaloupe ▶ Strawberries

▶ Honeydew ▶ Watermelon

▶ Kiwis

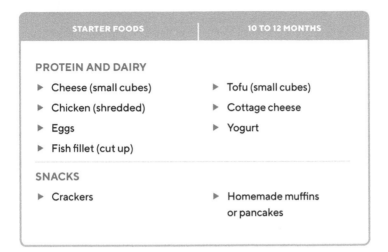

STARTER FOODS	10 TO 12 MONTHS

PROTEIN AND DAIRY

- ▶ Cheese (small cubes)
- ▶ Chicken (shredded)
- ▶ Eggs
- ▶ Fish fillet (cut up)

- ▶ Tofu (small cubes)
- ▶ Cottage cheese
- ▶ Yogurt

SNACKS

- ▶ Crackers

- ▶ Homemade muffins or pancakes

Learn and Play

PUSH THE CREATIVE BOUNDARY

If your kids aren't in childcare, and no one else at home or in the extended family (caretaker) has the time to push the creative envelope, this is your chance. Giving kids different mediums to express themselves will increase their dexterity and creativity. Join in the fun—play together, especially since some of these play elements (like water) require supervision anyway:

- ▶ Water-soluble markers

- ▶ Crayons (big fat ones are great for little hands)

- ▶ Puréed food art to explore the colors of foods: try green (peas), orange (sweet potatoes), and blue (blueberries). If they lick their fingers, all the better!

- ▶ Water and a sponge, water and spoons, water and anything

- ▶ Sensory/squishy bags (see page 69)

- ▶ Toy phone

- ▶ Workbench

HOW TO RUN A SUCCESSFUL PLAYDATE

Whether you are a stay-at-home dad or just taking the reins for Saturday morning, getting together with other parents and kids is an eventual must. If you're not in a hurry to do this, just remember that your baby's celebrating his first birthday this month. If he doesn't have a friend his age to invite, you'll at least want to start socializing him now so you're set up with a BFF for next year's party! Here are some tips for a successful playdate:

DON'T EXPECT INTERACTION. Babies tend to parallel play. This means they will sit next to each other and play without appearing to notice each other. But often they are watching and noticing. And eventually they will interact, likely by taking the toy out of the other baby's hands or mouth.

PLAN FOR AN HOUR. If you go to their home or they come to yours, an hour is plenty to start. Babies get overstimulated and tired, and so do dads. You don't want to be held hostage in a playdate where you realize your dad counterpart has nothing to say but does appear to be planning to stay the day. So call it an hour upfront.

ASK ABOUT THEIR EXPERIENCE. If you don't know how to break the ice, remember you're both parents. Pick other dads' brains about fatherhood. Ask for advice or suggestions on how to handle things you're dealing with.

MEET ON NEUTRAL GROUND. A great way to be able to keep playtime flexible is to meet at the playground. Everyone brings their own snacks and waters, and when baby cries, well, gotta go!

Clean

HOW TO ENCOURAGE A GOOD HELPER

Baby isn't ready to run the vacuum, but he can start understanding the concept of helping with simple tasks. These teach baby that everything has its place, and boosts confidence as you cheer him on for his efforts.

TOYS. Make a game out of it. Sing, talk, and sort as you and baby return toys to their proper place. If baby puts one in the bin, it's a victory!

WASHCLOTH. Wash your face! Wash your nose! Wash your feet! Of course, you will then need to really wash those things.

PUT THAT BACK PLEASE! Baby understands a *lot*. If baby responds to your request and puts the remote down, thank her and give her a kiss.

CAN I HAVE ONE? Ask baby to serve you one of her puffs—she might just pop it in your mouth. Reward this with a big "Thank you! What a good sharer!"

Sleep

HOW TO SLEEP TRAIN

Baby may begin to have separation anxiety when you or your partner aren't around. The stress of this can really rear its head at night, especially if baby's in his own room. With our kids, it made more sense for me to take the reins of sleep training. Full disclosure: We only did it with one kid and then threw it out the window. It's a tough gig—you'll feel guilty, tired, and impatient—but if you're expecting it, just know that it will become easier. Keep these things in mind:

GIVE IT AN HOUR. This dad advocates a peaceful wind-down or prelude. Set aside an hour or two before bedtime to feed him dinner and play lightly for a bit while food is digesting. Prepare a warm bath and get him into comfy pajamas. Lower the lights and read him a book while you rock together in a chair.

ESTABLISH A ROUTINE. If you continue to stick to something similar to what I've mentioned above, baby will begin to expect and anticipate what is happening next, like, *you're going to bed!*

ENLIST THE LOVEYS. By that, I mean find something that comforts them. Perhaps it's a wind-up plush or having Alexa play a lullaby on a timer. Maybe it's a smooth satin or silky piece of fabric that they like holding—our babies all had these small satin squares from Swaddle Designs that get Mom or Dad's scents on them by wearing them under your shirt for an hour . . . all four of our kids used these, and they work like magic.

REASSURE BABY. As you're laying her down, maybe this is a hand on her back for a few moments until she closes her eyes. It could be as extreme as what I went through with my son, Charlie. I used to have to lie on the floor next to his crib until he was asleep and then army crawl or move with ninja-like reflexes to sneak out of his room.

BE CONSISTENT. Consistency is key. It will get frustrating, having to continuously go in and out of their room at night, but stick with it—eventually it will start to take.

DON'T FEEL GUILTY. Baby will cry, but we made an effort *not* to run into the room at the first sign of them being upset—we always let them go just a few minutes. Almost always, they eventually self-soothed. I'll note that I was always watching them on the video monitor to make certain that their cries weren't from something like being pinched in the crib or having a leg stuck in the rails, etc.

HOW TO TRANSITION NAPTIME

Around this age, baby may begin dropping her morning nap. Or her afternoon nap—which is even trickier, because then she falls asleep at 5 p.m. and is then bright-eyed and ready to go at 3 in the morning. These are a few commonsense tips when naptime shifts occur.

LIMIT NAPTIME. If baby is falling asleep at an inopportune time, or the nap is going on too long, wake her up.

TRY TO TIME CAR RIDES OR STROLLER WALKS. These are like drugs to a baby—your baby will fall asleep no matter how loud you play the radio.

TRY TO KEEP IT CONSISTENT. Once you find a groove, try to stick with it.

WATCH FOR GOOD NIGHTTIME SLEEP. If baby's not napping to your liking, but sleeps well at night, you're out of luck. That's just your baby's way.

SHIFT BEDTIME. You can always try shifting baby's bedtime a little earlier or later. This might produce the nap you're looking for.

Learn and Play

HOW TO ENGAGE YOUR 10- TO 12-MONTH OLD

Your baby's development is greatly enhanced when you're interactive with them!

▶ Introduce hide-and-seek. Hide objects and let them find them—in your shirt, behind your back, just out of sight.

▶ Play Patty Cake or sooo big.

▶ Drape a sheet between two pieces of furniture to make baby's first clubhouse.

▶ Turn a large cardboard box into a tunnel by folding in both ends. Go to the other end and encourage baby to crawl through to you.

▶ Play "Where's the _____?" Ask baby "Where's my nose?" and see if she acknowledges it, either by looking, pointing, or touching. "Where's the dog?"

▶ Sort items into categories. Show him how all the blue blocks go here, all the red blocks go there.

▶ Turn off the TV. It's hard to compete when baby's distracted by the TV. Instead, play some music and sing along.

HOW TO BUILD CHILD'S LANGUAGE SKILLS

Help your baby to build her vocabulary and language skills. The ideas are endless, but here are a few.

JUST TALK. You always wanted to be a sports commentator, here's your shot—do play-by-plays, narrating everything that you're doing together. You might read him *The Wall Street Journal,* or you might be that parent who is always talking in a goofy voice to your kid, but who cares; either way it's building him up!

POINT THINGS OUT. Say, "There's the dog! Hi, Buddy!" Then later, "Where's the dog? Where's Buddy?" and see how baby reacts.

READ DIFFERENT BOOKS. She may have a favorite, but switch up your nightly routine and enjoy a variety of books. If you find that you're rushing your nighttime read, do it in the morning instead. And give her some board books to enjoy and chew on during the day.

FOLLOW BABY'S INTEREST. If something catches baby's eye, respond to it: "Oh, isn't that a pretty flower? That's a red one!"

Baby Gear

Must-Have

▶ **Safety bumpers:** If you have low tables, protect baby's head by surrounding hard corners of your furniture with soft bumpers.

▶ **Walking shoes:** If baby's getting close to walking, she'll need some shoes for walking! Get her properly sized for a good fit.

▶ **Sun gear:** Now that baby's moving beyond the safe confines of his covered stroller, protect him with a nice sun hat, sunglasses, and, of course, sunscreen.

▶ **Winter gear:** Depending on where you live, you may experience a long winter. Don't hide inside. Fresh air is awesome for baby in any season—just make sure baby is well protected with hat, gloves, snowsuit, etc. Babies should not be out in extreme cold, however (or extreme heat, for that matter).

Nice to Have

▶ **Snack cups:** A baby with a snack in hand is usually a pretty happy baby. Don't let baby get hangry—fill that little cup with puffs and be on your way.

▶ **Treaded socks:** These are great for baby to wear around the house to avoid slipping on hardwood floors or tile.

- **Pushing toys:** If baby is starting to get around, get a toy she can push around the room with great sound and visual effects.

- **A first ride-on toy:** Baby may not be able to get on or off, but you can push her around, or she can sit on it and enjoy the bells and whistles that come with it.

- **Jogging stroller:** This is the perfect age for a child to enjoy a quick ride around the neighborhood. He's got enough strength in his head and neck, and the constantly changing surroundings will take advantage of his increased ability to focus on something.

- **18-month outfits and beyond:** It's always a good idea to start shopping for kids clothes a size ahead of where they're at. And you've probably figured out by now that a 12-month-old is often wearing 18- or 24-month clothing. So whether it requires venturing out onto a shopping trip, tossing it out there as a gift idea for relatives, or accepting hand-me-downs from other parents, keep the closets stocked!

Pass

- **Fancy shoes:** What's the point?

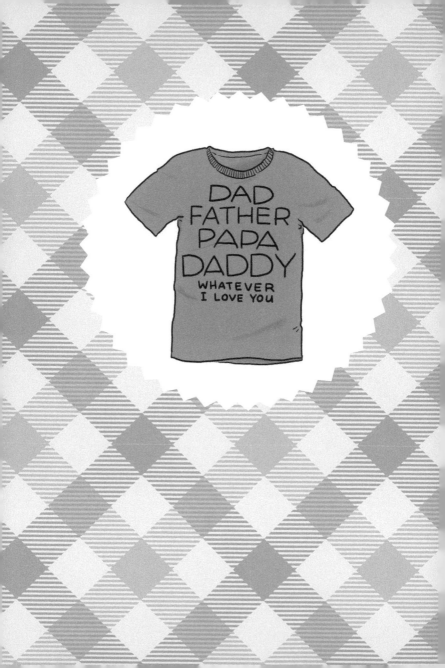

MONTH 10

AVERAGE SIZE	WEIGHT COMPARISON
19 pounds	Boombox

By the time this final quarter of the first year rolls around, you are probably getting ready to run a victory lap around the neighborhood. Month 10 means the only thing slowing down is the appetite. Baby is off to the races—crawling, possibly pulling herself up, and cruising. This kid is fully on the move and, quite frankly, it's borderline terrifying. It's an indication of what is right around the corner: *walking.*

The most essential piece of gear during this time is the baby jail. I doubt that we're the only parents to call it that, and if you're not familiar, it's an octagonal connecting gate enclosure. Think of it as something similar to the metal containment shell that Iron Man deployed to keep the Hulk in place while the Avengers were incapacitated. The goal is to keep superbaby in one place so you can actually go to the bathroom for 30 seconds without him making a run for it. Don't get me wrong, the ExerSaucer you probably bought a few months ago is exceptional, but baby will begin to get bored of the same toys day in and out. In fact, you may become an expert at the bait and switch: keeping some toys in the closet and then rotating them in and out to keep your little one happy. Baby is smart, and baby is fast. Just try and keep up.

BABY STATS

▶ Baby is sleeping an average of 10 to 12 hours per night.

▶ Taking two naps during the day, still 1½ to 2 hours.

▶ Baby is potentially banging his head on crib rails or walls—this is more common with boys than girls.

▶ Bottles or breast—total intake is somewhere between 24 and 30 ounces a day. With solids becoming more frequent, she is drinking less.

▶ Baby is eating ¼ to ½ cup each of grains, fruit and veggies, dairy and protein. These measurements can vary as long as your baby is gaining weight.

▶ Baby is beginning to use push toys.

▶ She may be able to use wider riding toys that are low to the ground like a fire truck or race car.

▶ Musical items are a big hit.

▶ At this point, you'll begin to be getting a sense of your baby's personality. Baby may have a few special items he's attached to—perhaps a stuffed animal or favorite book.

▶ Baby is pulling himself up from a seated position.

▶ Baby is squatting while holding stuff and able to sit back down.

▶ Baby should also be able to cruise, either by crawling/crab-walking or while hanging on to furniture and shuffling his feet.

▶ **Her pincer grasp (coordination of index finger to thumb) is almost mastered.**

    ▶ *Baby should be and will be grabbing almost anything in sight and putting it in her mouth. If you haven't already put the place on lockdown, get on it!*

    ▶ *Baby will begin to be able to fit smaller items into larger ones, such as stacking cups or plastic kitchen bowls.*

    ▶ *He is able to grasp a spoon and can probably almost use it to feed himself.*

    ▶ *Baby will begin to mimic behavior of those around them. If you're crying or upset, baby may show the same actions.*

    ▶ *Your little one may already know little phrases like "bye-bye," "dog" or "cat."*

    ▶ *She may be able to clap her hands.*

MOM STATS

▶ **If Mom is still breastfeeding, challenges may include pumping, rejection by baby, clogged ducts, or weaning.**

NOT-TO-MISS APPOINTMENTS

▶ **No scheduled pediatric appointments**

Goals

CRUISE DIRECTOR

Join a class. Consider looking into local parent-and-baby classes being offered, such as music, art, yoga, sensory play, or swimming. This is an opportunity for you to spend some quality time with your baby to explore new things. For me, it was an opportunity to get out of the house and meet other parents who were going through a similar stage in their child's development. Nothing is more comforting than hearing that other parents are having it worse than you! LOL.

PLAN AHEAD

Acknowledge behaviors. Behavior training can start now! It's never too early to begin calling attention to your baby's good behaviors or actions. Even if it's simple things like turning the pages of a book gently without ripping them or putting a stuffed animal back in the box instead of on the floor. **Apply positive reinforcement.** And in the same breath as we talk about positive reinforcement, it's also not a bad idea to begin to correct certain behaviors or actions. Your baby is beginning to be able to understand the word "no." You don't need to yell—your tone is the most effective indicator of your message. You can also physically correct what he's doing; for instance, putting books back in the bin or on the shelf. Maybe it's moving his hands away from the cable box after he has just turned off the finale of *Naked and Afraid*.

SELF-CARE

Join a parenting group. And it doesn't have to be one for just dads. Every time my wife and I have had to move since we've had kids (at least six times), I've had to start all over—meeting new friends and finding other kids for my kids to play with. Despite my occasional disdain for Facebook, the community aspect did afford me the opportunity to find some like-minded parents with the kids the same age. We took turns having one another over for an hour or two and alternated weeks. It was a good opportunity for our kids to work on their social skills (and me as well!). You never know what good things can come out of pushing your own comfort boundaries and meeting some new folks.

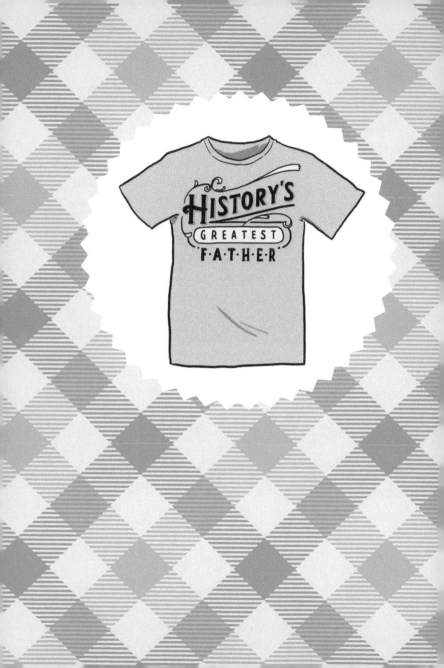

MONTH 11

AVERAGE SIZE	WEIGHT COMPARISON
19 pounds	Small car tire, empty golf bag

Now that baby is getting a bit older, he can understand "no." It doesn't mean he *likes* hearing it, but he can start to put two and two together and figure out that he should not be doing whatever activity is resulting in hearing that word. During this time, the baby will be starting to test his limits—and yours. Baby will decide that the best time for this is when he has had a massive diaper blowout and you're frantically trying to change him while he wiggles in and out of fecal matter on your new duvet cover. Just last week, I walked in to my wife changing Evelyn's diaper on the carpet using both bare feet on baby's shoulders to keep her secure as she expertly changed her diaper. Sometimes it takes all hands (and feet) on deck to get it done.

Along with maturing in a developmental sense, your little one is starting to thin out and potentially losing some of that baby chubbiness. They are beginning to graduate from baby to toddler very quickly. *Already?*

BABY STATS

▶ Baby is sleeping between 10 and 12 hours per night and taking two 1½- to 2-hour naps.

▶ Baby is nursing or bottle-feeding no more than three to four times a day.

▶ Baby is eating ¼ to ½ cup each of grains, fruit and veggies, dairy, and protein every day, through a combination of being fed and feeding self.

▶ Baby may have 3 to 4 ounces of juice (optional).

▶ Baby has a stronger sense of likes and dislikes and her attention span is growing.

▶ Baby is using emotions to get what he wants.

▶ Baby is cruising around on his feet by holding on to furniture, pulling open cabinets and drawers, and getting into everything, including things he shouldn't be.

▶ Baby is an escape artist, able to wriggle out of diapers, high chairs, and strollers. Always make sure she is properly buckled in.

▶ Baby is making verbal strides, beginning to accumulate words. Her number of spoken words is still low, but the number of words she understands could range from 20 to 50.

▶ Baby is beginning to point at things.

▶ Baby is playing with toys that encourage hand-eye coordination: blocks, stacking toys, puzzles, pegboards, bead mazes, and activity cubes.

MOM STATS

▶ If Mom is still breastfeeding, challenges may include pumping, rejection by baby, clogged ducts, or weaning.

NOT-TO-MISS APPOINTMENTS

▶ No scheduled pediatric appointments

Goals

CRUISE DIRECTOR

Plan a birthday party. It's coming up soon. What kind of party are you thinking? A dinner party with family, or a huge extravaganza with a rental inflatable bounce house? Have family flying in from out of state? Start working on that invitation list and preparing your home for the excitement.

SELF-CARE

Get ready for a toddler. Baby turning one is the beginning of toddlerhood. Are you ready for this? Back at the start of this year, you had dreams for the kind of father you wanted to be. Check back in with those—are you on the right path? Specifically, are you up physically for this very active next stage? If you could use some work here, start with a walk around the block. Bring your little buddy—they'll appreciate it!

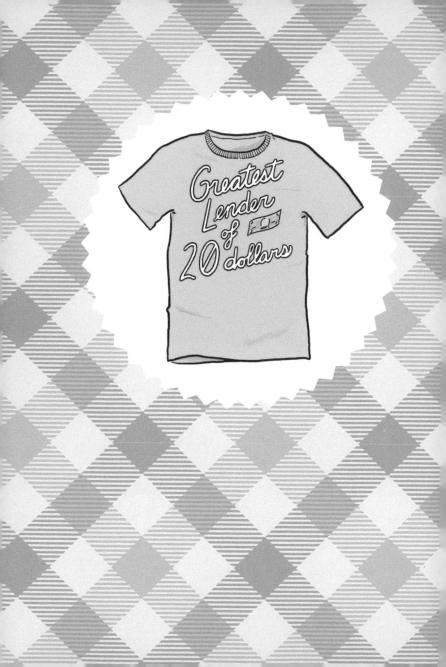

MONTH 12

AVERAGE SIZE	WEIGHT COMPARISON
20 to 21 pounds	Propane tank for a gas grill, bag of sand

Happy Dadiversary!

By this month, games have become a way of life. We live on a golf course, and every day, Evelyn and I walk and pick up golf balls that have sliced into our back yard. We've got a basket of 500 or more at this point, and Evie's favorite game is to pull herself up to the basket, and drop them onto the hardwood floor, one by one.

Babies also start to learn about sequences. They begin realizing that to accomplish their goals, they need to follow tasks in a certain order. For example, baby might recognize that to eat cereal (not that they're feeding themselves adequately with a spoon yet), he would need to dip the spoon into the bowl before putting it into his mouth.

This month is one of the most emotional for me—you've made it through the year. We've always thrown big first-birthday parties for all of our family friends, because it's a huge milestone celebration. And, as much as it's a party for her to have her very own "smash cake" (hint: many grocery store chains will gift you a *free* one on baby's first birthday), and for you to get those killer frosting-covered photos, it's also a celebration for you and your partner. You're graduating into the toddler stage. What a year.

BABY STATS

▶ Baby is sleeping around 10 to 12 hours a night.

▶ Baby is having two daytime naps (possibly cutting one out to ensure better nighttime sleep).

▶ Baby's total sleep is between 12 and 14 hours.

▶ Nursing or formula tops out around 24 ounces.

▶ Baby is eating ¼ to ½ cup or more of grains, fruit and veggies, dairy, and protein daily.

▶ Baby may be drinking 3 to 4 ounces of juice (optional).

▶ Baby is walking or almost walking.

▶ Baby is pushing and pulling toys throughout the house.

▶ You may notice a drop in appetite.

▶ Your baby's weight has likely tripled since birth.

▶ Baby has grown between 9 to 11 inches. This is almost a 50 percent increase since birth.

▶ Baby's brain is around 60 percent the size of an adult's.

▶ Baby is eating with fingers and achieving continued mastery of the spoon.

▶ Baby is able to help parents while getting dressed, such as putting arms or legs where they need to go.

▶ Baby is using different items properly, like a spoon, phone, or hairbrush.

▶ At this point, it's okay to make the transition from breast milk to regular cow's milk, however, don't use low-fat milk until after his second birthday.

▶ Baby has an increased vocabulary and is probably saying a few words like "Mama," "Dada," "no," "uh-oh," and "bye-bye."

▶ Baby is testing her limits; for instance, going up the stairs, seeing how much food she can throw on the floor before you correct her, and getting into things previously unexplored.

NOT-TO-MISS APPOINTMENTS

▶ 1-year appointment: Check stats from your 9-month appointment and consult with your pediatrician to make sure that everything is within the acceptable range for development. A few things that your doctor may be looking for:

  ▶ *Baby's weight, length, and head circumference*
  ▶ *Overall physical exam*
  ▶ *Potential vaccine for measles, mumps, rubella, chicken pox, or another (booster) shot of something already received*
  ▶ *If it's fall or winter, a flu shot may be recommended*
  ▶ *Is baby pulling up? Standing? Walking?*
  ▶ *Has baby started talking yet? What words is he using?*
  ▶ *How is baby handling eating solid foods?*
  ▶ *Does baby use both hands for everything?*
  ▶ *Does baby point at things?*

Goals

CRUISE DIRECTOR

Host that first-birthday party. The first-birthday party is a *big* one. My wife always went off on these, but they seemed to be more for the parents than the actual kid. However, it's a great time to celebrate, and it's something they won't remember, so memorialize it with lots of photos—to be able to look back on pictures when they're older will provide lots of entertainment.

STAFF MEETING

Reminisce and document. When was the last time you wrote something in their baby book? Together with your partner, take an hour and jot some of the funny or memorable stories down before they get lost in the archives of your memory.

BONDING TIME

Plan another party, for two. You did this first year together, and you should celebrate your achievements, great and small. Surprise your tag team partner with a night they'll never forget.

DADDY DOULA

Support Mom if she considers weaning. Get baby to use other sources of food. Cut back on breastfeeding. You could also consider buying Mr. Milker, so you can breastfeed too—or not.

Conclusion

Nothing has impacted my existence more than watching my kids make their debut into the world. Each and every pregnancy has been different—a roller coaster of emotional, physical, and mental challenges. But there's nothing that warms the heart and soul more than your own little one looking up to you with those beautiful eyes.

If you read the first book in this series, *We're Pregnant! The First-Time Dad's Pregnancy Handbook* or follow my blog, *Dad or Alive*, I first want to thank you for your loyalty. Beyond that, you'll know that while I've been tagged as an expert here and there from different publications, I am just a regular guy trying to be the best dad that I can be.

I don't have all the answers, nor have I ever represented myself as someone who does. I research and listen to recommendations that are offered by accredited agencies and licensed physicians, but at the end of the day, everyone's situation is different, and I often find the intersection between internal instinct and common sense to reach the best decision.

The first year of fatherhood is a blessing. With every blowout diaper or grocery store tantrum comes a "first." The first time they crawl, the first time you hear their voice as they say their first word, that first tooth, the first time they clap their hands, and the moment they take their first steps and get turned loose on the world (and your hopefully babyproofed home).

This book was meant as not only a crutch, but also a blueprint to encourage you to be the best partner and dad to your little one.

With Ava, Charlie, Mason, and Evelyn, I've often found myself groaning to veteran parents about how "I'm in the thick of it right now" and that they are on the other side with older children. Their response is ALWAYS the same. Childhood is but a fleeting moment and, before you know it, they'll be grown and gone. Someday your home will once again be silent; someday the toys will be gone. Cherish every day, no matter how stressful life may get. Stop, take a deep breath, and recognize the joy in being part of their lives. In child-rearing, there was never a truer statement: the days are long, but the years are ungodly short.

Parenthood is a bumpy road, but your baby is glad to be traveling that road with you ...

Glossary

baby blues: the mood swings, excessive crying, and/or worrying a mother may experience for about two weeks after birth; if Mom continues to experience these feelings, she might be dealing with a postpartum mood disorder such as postpartum depression or postpartum anxiety

babyproofing: removing or containing small and/or dangerous items throughout the home to keep them away from your little one; also called "childproofing"

colic: a term used to describe when a generally healthy, well-fed infant cries by the "rule of threes": more than three hours a day, three or more days a week, for longer than three weeks

colostrum: a protein- and antibody-rich fluid produced by Mom's breasts before they actually produce milk that provides the necessary nourishment during those first precious days after birth

cradle cap: a flaky, reddish rash that has a scaly appearance to it and may look like dandruff

doula: a nonmedical professional who doesn't deliver babies or provide any type of medical care; however, if certified, a doula has taken a training program/exam on how to help pregnant women and their families during the course of pregnancy

eczema: a condition that causes an itchy, red skin irritation; while it can occur in adults, it's also common in children

envelope neck: the folded neckline on a onesie that can be pulled down over the baby instead of up; lifesaver in the event of a poop blowout

essential oils: concentrated oils in various scents that can be diffused into the air that may contain healing properties; consult with your pediatrician before applying to your kid's skin

Family and Medical Leave Act (FMLA): a U.S. labor law requiring covered employers to provide employees with unpaid leave, as well as time off, with their jobs being protected

fontanel: a developing area on the top of the head of your little one; often called a "soft spot"

lactation consultant: a health care professional specializing in the clinical management of breastfeeding who helps women experiencing breastfeeding problems, such as latching difficulties, painful nursing, and/or low milk production, as well as assists in self-care and management techniques related to the breastfeeding journey

meconium: your baby's first stool, a black, viscous, tar-like combination of materials ingested during baby's time in the uterus—hardly recognizable as feces

night nurse: a nurse hired to take care of your baby at night, so you're able to get some sleep

nursing blisters: tiny, white blisters that form over the opening of the milk duct on the nipple

pacifier: a silicone nipple with a mouth shield and handle or ring used to soothe an infant, also known as a "binky" and "teether"; using it can be a difficult habit for toddlers to break

plugged ducts: hard, localized, tender lumps that block the flow of breast milk, often caused by an internal obstruction within a milk duct inside the breast; also called "blocked ducts" or "clogged ducts"

postpartum mood disorders: include common, temporary, and treatable postpartum anxiety (PPA) and postpartum depression (PPD) that ride along with childbirth; although both Mom and Dad can experience them, Mom is at highest risk; symptoms may include extreme sadness, excessive crying, anxiousness, inability to make decisions or think clearly, and insomnia/inability to sleep, among others

probiotics: live microorganisms that typically improve gut flora and provide certain health benefits when ingested; generally safe to consume

sensory play: play that stimulates your child's senses: sight, smell, taste, touch, and hearing

SIDS (sudden infant death syndrome): the sudden, unexplained death of an infant; it's rare and generally happens at night, leading to the name "crib death"

swaddle: wrapping your baby up "like a burrito" to soothe her; the constricted movement and tightness may remind her of the womb

thrush: a type of yeast infection in the mouth, which can also be found on other parts of the body and can be responsible for diaper rash

tummy time: placing baby on his stomach, starting around three months old, for up to 30 minutes a day to help him build strength to eventually flip over and ultimately sit up

weaning: stopping breastfeeding

Resources

For Fathers

All Pro Dad (AllProDad.com): This site offers support ranging from daily one-minute encouragement emails to interactive sports experiences.

City Dads Group (CityDadsGroup.com): This group brings dads together through meetups, podcasts, boot camps, and social media.

The Dad (TheDad.com): Here you'll find jokes, memes, parenting humor, and "kind, involved fathers who talk like real people."

The Dad 2.0 Summit (Dad2Summit.com): The summit is an annual gathering for "understanding and connecting with modern men" who "see fatherhood as a vital social good."

Dad or Alive (DadorAlive.com): My blog houses confessions of an unexpected stay-at-home dad and talks about everything from the ages and stages of development to what happens when Dad's in deep shit!

Daddy Style Diaries (DaddyStyleDiaries.com): This lifestyle blog is focused on fatherhood, travel, and cars.

Designer Daddy (DesignerDaddy.com): Here you'll find discussions of parenthood and fatherhood from the gay dad of an adopted son, as well as crafting projects and pop culture references.

Fatherly (Fatherly.com): This leading digital fatherhood brand seeks to "empower men to raise great kids and lead more fulfilling adult lives" through original content.

How to Be a Dad (HowToBeADad.com): This blog offers a humorous take on fatherhood and provides "you're not alone" support.

Life of Dad (LifeOfDad.com): From shows, podcasts, and even DadTV, Life of Dad provides advice on everything from gear to date night.

Lunchbox Dad (LunchboxDad.com): This site focuses on making lunchtime fun, offering ideas for bento box lunches, parenting articles, and product reviews.

Mr. Dad (MrDad.com): This site offers advice for every type, stage, and role of fatherhood, as well as product reviews and podcasts.

National At-Home Dad Network (AtHomeDad.org): Here you can find "advocacy, community, education, and support" for primary caregiving dads.

National Fatherhood Initiative (Fatherhood.org): NFI is the "nation's leading non-profit organization working to end father absence," and has partnered with the Armed Services, the Department of Justice, and community and charitable organizations like the Salvation Army.

National Center for Fathering (Fathers.com): Here you'll find training, research, and even a Fathering Library designed to provide support, encouragement, and guidance.

Tales from the Poop Deck (TalesFromThePoopDeck.com): This cleverly titled blog discusses "navigating the stormy waters of fatherhood."

General Parenting

Babble (Babble.com): This site, courtesy of Disney, covers everything from pregnancy and parenthood to entertainment and lifestyle topics.

BabyCenter (BabyCenter.com): As the "world's number one digital parenting resource," BabyCenter reaches more than 100 million people each month and offers content in nine different languages.

The *Huffington Post*—Parenting (HuffPost.com/life/parents): This branch of the *Huffington Post* offers modern parenting news and stories.

Parenting (Parenting.com): From stroller shopping to toddler activities to fertility planning, *Parenting* offers guidance for nearly every step of the journey.

Parents (Parents.com): Here you'll find access to all the resources from *Parenting* magazine, as well its other publications: Fit Pregnancy and Baby, Family Fun, Parents Latina, and Ser Padres.

Very Well Family (VeryWellFamily.com): Offering a "realistic and friendly approach to pregnancy and parenting," this site has content from health care professionals about pregnancy and parenting.

WebMD (WebMD.com): A go-to online resource for medical information. Ensure you discuss all symptoms and medical issues with your physician.

What to Expect (WhatToExpect.com): What to Expect combines medically reviewed health content, lighthearted discussions, and helpful planning information to "support happy, healthy pregnancies and happy, healthy babies."

For Loss, Depression, Coping, and Parent Care

Healing Hearts, Baby Loss Comfort (BabyLossComfort.com/grief): A comprehensive collection of sites and resources (including films, Facebook pages, and children's books) are offered here for anyone affected by the loss of a child.

National Suicide Prevention Lifeline (1-800-273-TALK / 1-800-273-8255 or use their webchat on suicidepreventionlifeline.org/chat): Free and confidential support for anyone in distress and resources for professionals and loved ones.

Postpartum Dads (PostpartumDads.org): Resources, information, and firsthand guidance are offered through this website for families dealing with postpartum depression.

Postpartum Progress (PostpartumProgress.com): This site is "the world's most widely-read blog dedicated to maternal mental illness" and offers resources and support for parents dealing with postpartum- and pregnancy-related mental illnesses.

Postpartum Support International (Postpartum.net): PSI's mission is to increase awareness of postpartum-related emotional and mental changes among public and professional communities. Please note that their helpline doesn't handle emergencies.

Share: Pregnancy and Infant Loss Support (NationalShare.org): This national community is for anyone—parents, loved ones, caregivers, and professionals—who has experienced the tragic loss of a baby.

References

American Academy of Pediatrics, Steven Shelov, P., MD, MS, FAAP, and Tanya Remer Altmann, MD, FAAP. *Caring for Your Baby and Young Child: Birth to Age 5.* New York: Bantam, 2009.

Brott, Armin A. *The New Father: A Dad's Guide to the First Year (3rd ed.).* New York: Abbeville Press, 2015.

Brown, Ari, and Denise Fields. *Baby 411: Clear Answers and Smart Advice for Your Baby's First Year (8th ed.).* Boulder, Colorado: Windsor Peak Press, 2017.

Dais, Dawn. *The Sh!t No One Tells You: A Guide to Surviving Your Baby's First Year.* New York: Seal Press, 2013.

Greenberg, Gary, and Jeannie Hayden. *Be Prepared: A Practical Handbook for New Dads.* New York: Simon & Schuster, 2004.

Hargis, Aubrey. *Baby's First Year Milestones: Promote and Celebrate Your Baby's Development with Monthly Games and Activities.* Berkeley, California: Rockridge Press, 2018.

Murkoff, Heidi, and Sharon Mazel. *What to Expect the First Year (3rd ed.).* New York: Workman Publishing Company, 2014.

Index

Acknowledgments

I've been fortunate enough to have been blessed with a wife and partner in a relationship that allows us to support one another's dreams, pick each other up after we've fallen, and find solace in sorrow.

We've shared four pregnancies together, as well as a fifth that was cut short with the heartache of a miscarriage. I wouldn't be half the man that I am today without my wife, Jen, and my kids—Ava, Charlie, Mason, and Evelyn—and the experiences we've endured together as a family.

Much love to my parents and siblings, Bruce, Joan, Eric, and Travis, as well as my parents-in-law, Bob and Elaine, and Jen's siblings and their partners, who have always welcomed me with open arms, love, and support (and made me an uncle seven times already!).

About the Author

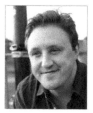 **Adrian Kulp** has worked as a comedy booking agent for CBS late-night television, a TV executive for Adam Sandler's Happy Madison Productions (*Rules of Engagement, The Goldbergs*) and as a vice president of development for Chelsea Handler's Borderline Amazing Productions (*After Lately, Comedians of Chelsea Lately*).

For the past nine years, he's been the voice behind the popular dad blog turned parenting memoir, *Dad or Alive: Confessions of an Unexpected Stay-at-Home Dad*. He's produced the reality series *Modern Dads* for A&E Networks, is a former contributor to *HuffPost*, *The Bump*, *Kids in the House*, and *Parents* magazine. He's also a partner at the largest online fatherhood community, Life of Dad, where he works on the creative team and heads branded content.

In 2018, he wrote the prequel to the book you're reading right now . . . *We're Pregnant! The First-Time Dad's Pregnancy Handbook*.

FUN FACT: Kulp wrote the prequel while he and his wife were going through their last pregnancy *and* finished this book just before that little baby turned one.

After 21 years in Pennsylvania, 14 years in Los Angeles, 5 years in Maryland, and 3 years in coastal Virginia, he's recently moved to Nashville, Tennessee, with his wife, Jen, and their four kids, Ava, Charlie, Mason, and Evelyn.

CPSIA information can be obtained
at www.ICGtesting.com
Printed in the USA
LVHW070309171121
703573LV00018B/1460

9 781641 524155